THERAPEUTIC RECREATION
FOR LONG-TERM CARE FACILITIES

THERAPEUTIC RECREATION FOR LONG-TERM CARE FACILITIES

Fred S. Greenblatt, M.S., CTRS
Activities Consultant
Director of Activities
The Jewish Home and Hospital for Aged
Kingsbridge Center
Bronx, New York

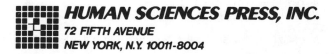
HUMAN SCIENCES PRESS, INC.
72 FIFTH AVENUE
NEW YORK, N.Y. 10011-8004

Copyright © 1988 by Human Sciences Press, Inc.
72 Fifth Avenue, New York, New York 10011

Printed in the United States of America
987654321

Library of Congress Cataloging-in-Publication Data
Greenblatt, Fred S.
  Therapeutic recreation for long-term care
facilities.

  Bibliography: p.
  Includes index.
  1. Recreational therapy for the aged.   2. Long-term
care facilities—Recreational activities.   I. Title.
[DNLM: 1. Geriatrics.   2. Long Term Care.   3. Recrea-
tion. WT 30 G798t]
RC953.8.R43G74   1987   615.8′5153′0880565   86-27697
ISBN 0-89885-356-7

*The Art of Writing
is the
Joy of Learning.*

This book is dedicated to the elderly, who have taught me through their significant contribution to the quality of life,

and to

my wife, Marge, and three sons, Scott, Russell, and Bryan, whose love and support have encouraged me to share all I have learned.

CONTENTS

PREFACE

The needs of today's elderly population have been increasingly addressed through the provision of higher standards of medical care both in the community and in the long-term care facility. However, the psychological and emotional needs of this minority still need to be recognized to a much larger extent.

Admission to a long-term care facility often highlights the losses experienced by the aged person, including his physical ability to function independently or his emotional need to feel like a worthwhile, total individual.

> Admission to a Nursing Home, no matter how good the facility may be, unfortunately adds to the old person's losses. Individuality and independence becomes difficult to achieve. The life of a Nursing Home person becomes fragmented. Old people in many instances are almost forced to sit back while dietary provides their food, housekeeping changes their linens and the nursing department gives them their medication, to name only a few ills. The physicians often treat their ailments, ignoring their psychological and emotional needs to be seen as a whole person. Professionals in the field of Geriatrics and Gerontology are witness to the effects of these physical and psychological losses on a daily basis. Growing old in America and becoming a Nursing Home patient should not parallel the end of a meaningful life.[1]

Once the daily needs (medical, nursing, dietary, etc.) of the client are met, a large block of unrestricted time becomes available. It then becomes the responsibility of the Activities department to satisfy the remaining psychological, emotional and social needs with a meaningful delivery of Therapeutic Recreation services.

The importance of a sound developmental, imaginative and well balanced activity program in a long-term care facility cannot be underestimated. However, providing the population of long-term care facilities with an appropriate and worthwhile program of activities is not an easy task. Through my years of experience as Activity Director, consultant and teacher, I continue to hear the cries of activity professionals and college students who seek assistance in learning to organize and implement successful therapeutic recreation services.

Although there are several books available which deal with the delivery of Therapeutic Recreation Service, much of the literature deals in a generalized manner with settings *other than* long-term care facilities and nursing homes. The information presented here will be applicable to all long-term care facilities. However, due to my extensive experience in nursing home settings, this will be the primary focus of the chapters to follow.

Many books on therapeutic recreation offer sound principles and techniques for general use with therapeutic recreation. However, the successful application of these principles and procedures related specifically to the activities programs of long-term care facilities become the responsibility of the reader. Unfortunately, the readers of such texts are usually those looking for the assistance required to design, organize and implement a recreation program in the long-term care facility or nursing home.

This book will provide its reader with a solid foundation of the principles and procedures of therapeutic recreation services. Of equal importance is the methodology utilized in applying these principles to a successful recreation program. Drawing upon the most current literature and research as well as my firsthand experience in the recreation profession, I have incorporated all aspects of therapeutic recreation necessary to the development and implementation of a well balanced activity program. The real issues and concerns affecting the recreation needs of the long-term care client and nursing home patient are identified and analyzed.

I have made this a comprehensive text by including areas which go beyond the initial theory and process of therapeutic recreation programming. Areas overlooked by other texts but which are equally significant to long-term care recreation programming are developed in each chapter.

Chapter One, "Understanding Therapeutic Recreation," offers a basis for understanding the terms "Recreation" and "Therapeutic Recreation." Inherent in these definitions is an examination of the principles and techniques which are recognized as essential elements in designing and implementing a successful therapeutic recreation program.

Chapter Two, "Therapeutic Recreation: Historical Implications," traces the origins of the recreation movement and examines its importance to the delivery of service to the ill and disabled population of the United States.

The need for a well defined philosophy and goal is essential not only in designing a well balanced program, but for the formation of therapeutic recreation as a profession and occupation as well. Chapter Three, "Developing a Philosophy and Goal," examines the current philosophy statement of the National Therapeutic Recreation Society (NTRS) and the significance of the leisure ability approach to the delivery of therapeutic recreation services. Developing a personal philosophy and goal necessary for the implementation of therapeutic recreation services is also examined.

With a basic understanding of therapeutic recreation and the development of a goal and philosophy, Chapter Four will provide an in depth examination of developing a well balanced program. A variety of methods and approaches will be reviewed including their implications to the program design and planning. Certain factors must be considered regardless of the method or approach utilized to design a program. A detailed evaluation of these elements is provided including assessment of the client's background (education, religious practices, socio-economic status, occupation, age related factors and disabilities), the agency's background (history, regulatory standards, organizational structure, staff facilities, equipment, budget, etc.), and available community resources (schools, churches, etc.).

Selecting appropriate activities is an integral part of the program planning process. Chapter Five will examine the behavioral factors effecting program design. Impairments in the behavioral areas (physical, cognitive, and affective) and their effect upon activity participation are discussed. Social interactive structures necessary for successful participation are also identified. Finally, activity adaptation is reviewed along with suggestions for types of activities.

The painstaking effort used to develop a well balanced program merits evaluation of that program. Evaluation plays a crucial role to the success of the program. Without it, there will be no way of increasing effectiveness of the program. Chapter Six, "Program Evaluation," will define evaluation and its process and will offer models, approaches and procedures for evaluation. Finally, the areas needed for evaluation will be identified.

Leadership in recreation is probably one of the most important ingredients of the well balanced program. Without a competent professional recreation leader the program will be inoperable regardless of all its assets and resources. Chapter Seven, "The Use of Effective Leadership," will examine leadership theories and styles, and its meaning and implications for effective programming. The nature and role of the leader including the activity director, supervisor and recreation leader will be addressed. Finally, understanding group dynamics and techniques for leadership of groups will be provided.

As a treatment modality with the cognitively impaired elderly, therapeutic recreation offers many advantages not shared by other interventions. First, it avoids the sense of threat which can accompany some of the more clinical modalities; secondly, it is presented as part of a familiar pattern of preferences; thirdly, it permits structure without regimentation. These three elements are very important for working with the cognitively impaired elderly.

Major goals for therapeutic recreation with these patients will be the focus of Chapter Eight. "Recreation for the Cognitively Impaired," will include specific activities found to be effective for working with this population of elderly, and the rationale for the use of these activities. Special problems to be anticipated in working with this population will also be documented.

The utilization of volunteer services in recreation programs cannot be overlooked. Budget cuts and the need for increased volunteer resources make the significance of their contribution to recreation programming more important than ever before.

Many activity directors wear two hats; that of director and that of volunteer director. Chapter Nine will delineate the values of volunteer services in recreation. Development of volunteer services including selection of a director, his role, and legal considerations will be examined. Orientation, training and interview methods will be discussed as well as areas of volunteer work and recognition needs.

Although documentation in therapeutic recreation is an essential function of professional services, activity personnel are continually faced with the increased burden of the paper work dilemma. Chapter Ten, "The Paper Work Dilemma," will examine documentation needs which go beyond resident care plans, including procedure manuals, attendance statistics, progress reports, file and audit systems and other paper work pertinent to the successful operation of the activity department. Writing effective care plans for individual client documentation will also be addressed.

Finally, the appendices will provide a wealth of resources including suggested activities and forms commonly used for the activity department.

The growth of our profession is dependent upon the sharing of ideas, philosophies and knowledge which effects the way in which we deliver therapeutic recreation services. This college level text will provide its reader with a comprehensive book to be utilized in understanding, developing and implementing the delivery of therapeutic recreation services. It is hoped that college students and instructors will use this text as a resource for therapeutic recreation and aging. It may also be referred to as a supplementary text for the related human sciences including courses in social work, recreation, leisure and physical education. It will also provide a "hands on" text for the recreation college intern and long-term care personnel such as the administrator, social worker, nurse, volunteer, and recreation leader and director. This book attempts to provide information which will help further the growth and progress of our profession and occupation.

Fred S. Greenblatt

ACKNOWLEDGMENTS

I would like to acknowledge with grateful thanks and appreciation the following people whose wisdom, support and guidance have helped turn my thoughts into the pages of this book.

First, to Harvey Finkelstein, Administrator, and Helene Meyers, Associate Administrator, of The Jewish Home and Hospital for Aged, Bronx, New York, whose commitment to the care of the elderly has fostered an environment within the long-term care facility conducive to the growth of their staff both professionally and personally.

To Ken Sherman, friend, colleague and Administrator, Central House, The Jewish Home and Hospital for Aged, New York City, whose unique administrative abilities, ardent support and belief in the significance of creative programming serve as an inspiration to the delivery of therapeutic recreation services.

To my wonderful staff, whose talent, skills and enthusiastic spirit are the essential ingredients to the success of our recreation programs.

To Dr. Miriam Lahey, friend and colleague, whose knowledge, guidance and untiring patience were instrumental to the completion of this book.

Finally, to Lucille Esralew, friend and colleague, whose expertise was instrumental to the implementation and success of the Pilot Program at The Jewish Home and Hospital for Aged.

I would also like to acknowledge the following for permission to use material which has contributed to the publishing of this book.

To Dr. Lahey for her significant contribution in writing "Recreation for the Cognitively Impaired," which is used with her permission as Chapter Eight.

Chapter 1

UNDERSTANDING THERAPEUTIC RECREATION

DEFINING RECREATION

Before we can begin to understand the process of therapeutic recreation, we must describe what we mean by the term "recreation." Recreation implies a variety of meanings and may be viewed in different contexts by the recreation professional.

Recreation and Leisure

The ability to enjoy "recreation" and its concomitant effects will depend upon one's leisure lifestyle. Leisure is seen as any block of free time. How we fill this free time becomes indicative of the values and attitudes we develop throughout our lifetime. Our daily experiences and relationships with family, education, occupation and religion establish certain attitudes and values which result in behaviors which comprise our leisure lifestyle.

Man's leisure time is directly related to work. The more time he works, the less time he has to spend on leisure. Thus, the pre-industrial American society demanded that man spend the majority of his time in work-related tasks. This was made necessary by the collective economic needs of the time as well as the individual's need to survive. As a result, leisure time spent in pleasurable recreation was viewed upon negatively by society.

Today's postwar industrial society has changed the philosophical basis of man's primary need to work. Increased technological advances have lead to increased leisure time resulting in the development of a more active recreation pattern and leisure lifestyle. In addition, retirement at earlier ages is creating a greater awareness of leisure time.

The continued growth of automation, computerization and leisure time will certainly result in the need for constructive, organized forms of recreation. Thus, recreation behavior and patterns of recreation are becoming a great deal more sophisticated. As Richard Kraus suggests, one of the underlying elements regarding the concern about recreation in modern America includes:

> the dramatic expansion of leisure (unobligated time) that has come about as a consequence of industrialization and automation, the shorter work week, earlier retirement, medical and social advances and modern technology in general.[1]

In spite of the advances of the post-industrial society, one needs to be reminded that the economic situation still largely determines the amount of leisure time one has available to him. In addition to the time element involved, one's social class will determine how one's leisure time is spent. Thus, studies have shown that those of the lower class need to spend more time working and less time in leisure pursuits.

The concepts of leisure and recreation are therefore highly related. As James Murphy indicates, "leisure is a time of a special kind: recreation is activity (or inactivity) of special kinds. Recreation takes place during leisure; but not all leisure is given over to recreation."[2]

The relationship between leisure and recreation is a philosophy of values and ideals. These beliefs, attitudes and behaviors become the basis for recreation patterns used to create one's leisure lifestyle.

Viewing Recreation As an Experience

Professionals also view recreation as an experience one takes on while engaging in a particular activity during one's leisure time. This activity may be anything which represents pleasure or enjoyment, relaxation or a disconnection from any of life's pressures. A recreation experience is usually characterized as an experience which has no specific goal other than pleasure itself. The time it takes to participate in this recreation experience may vary. One may choose to participate in a sport for an hour while others may experience the pleasure of a two-week vacation.

Recreation is a personalized, individualized experience. As J. Tillman Hall points out:

> the cause or motivating factors for recreation may not be the same for any two people and they vary from time to time for the same individual. One person may be seeking physical exercise while another seeks companionship. One theory may adequately cover the motivating cause for

recreation during one hour, while an entirely different theory may describe the drives which stimulate the same activity at a later time. The motivating cause may not be evident to even the participant.[3]

Thus, recreation for one may not be recreation for someone else. For example, the sewing of garments by a professional seamstress may not have the same value as that obtained by the resident who experiences pleasure and joy from completing a dress in a recreational sewing class. Recreation is a personal experience which differs for every one of us. It therefore becomes an internal experience, characterized by the fact that the person is totally aware of his involvement in this recreation experience.

Viewing Recreation As a Social Institution

The developing values and attitudes toward leisure and the pattern of recreation behavior necessitates the availability of leisure and recreation services. These services are provided through a network of social institutions.

Leisure and recreation services will be determined by the people they serve. Thus, the need for these services will differ according to one's occupation, social class, race and ethnic backgrounds.

Many studies have been done to determine the use of leisure upon class differences. In a study by Clye R. White,[4] several categories of leisure were identified. These included:

Public recreation facilities

Group work agencies

Church

Museums

Libraries

Commercial amusements

This study indicated that lower classes used public facilities more often than upper classes, and that the home was the most used setting for leisure involvement.

The social factors affecting the recreation movement were of great importance following World War II. The large majority of the white middle class began moving to the surburban areas of the cities. This move toward suburbia spurred the growth of new schools as well as social institutions which could provide the new population with appropriate leisure services and recreation activities.

On the other hand, the cities became the home of either the poor or the wealthy. This created a new set of demands for recreation activities and leisure services which would satisfy the need of a new population including minority groups.

As a social institution, Avedon explains, "it is a formal structure and apparatus that includes social functionaries (personnel) who through the structure attempt to serve the needs of society."[5]

Recreation has become a social institution through a system of organized services which various sectors of the population have demanded. Through the social structure of institutions a vareity of recreation services are offered to the population at large. Social institutions vary depending upon the type of people who utilize their facilities. For example, one may find museums or zoos in certain areas of the country while these same areas may lack community centers or other resources.

Because of the wide variety of recreation needs of today's society, socia' institutions vary in structure and purpose. Institutions such as hospital and nursing homes provide recreation services through social structures However, the primary objective of their recreation service is not to achieve a purely pleasurable experience, but to offer recreation as a therapeutic intervention, thereby achieving a means to an end.

Thus, even through social institutions, one can see that the term "recreation" begins to take on different meanings for different people.

Viewing Recreation As a Service

Through the social institution comes recreation services. These services are offered in a variety of ways to a variety of groups. Due to the multitude of recreation services, those who provide them must be properly educated and trained to carry out the service required.

Avedon points to the primary recreation service elements as:

   Administrative
   Supervisory
   Leadership
   Consultative
   Coordinative
   Research[6]

An understanding of the role of these service elements as they relate to the long-term care facility is necessary for the program planner. Further, an understanding of their relationship within the social institution or nursing home will provide for more efficient program planning.

Because of the importance of the recreation service elements of the long-term care facility, these will be dealt with in detail in a later chapter.

Within the social institution, such as the long-term care facility, recreation services are provided with the goals or objectives of the institution at hand. The goals and objectives of the activities department must be carried out through a network of services which parallel the overall philosophy and goals of the institution.

In addition to the primary recreation service elements, the staffs of other departments play an equal role in satisfying resident needs. Often, the services of these departments must be coordinated to provide the achievement of goals within the philosophical framework of the institution. The use of auxiliary staff services within the recreation department will also be discussed in a later chapter.

Whatever services are offered, the goal or objective of the social institution should be clear. Thus, based upon the needs of the social institution, the goals of the recreation service may be established. One must therefore be aware of the needs of each particular patient or client for whom he is providing his recreation service.

Based upon an understanding of the characteristics of the term "recreation," we may now begin to examine more closely what we mean by the term "therapeutic recreation."

DEFINING THERAPEUTIC RECREATION

Recreation and Rehabilitation

What is therapeutic recreation? Unfortunately, the answer is not as simple as adding two plus two. Although the result may in fact equal four, the approach utilized in reaching the answer is as important as the answer itself.

The use of certain principles, techniques and processes add up to an understanding of therapeutic recreation. However, it is how these principles and theories are utilized that leads to a definition of therapeutic recreation.

All recreation professionals will agree that therapeutic recreation is one specific area which the field of recreation encompasses. A major goal of this service is to help maximize the total functional ability of its client. Through its therapeutic intervention it becomes a helping process concerned with alleviating humanistic problems related to psychological and physical disability. Therapeutic recreation cannot be considered a cure in itself, but it helps bring about a rehabilitation of the *total person* through its therapeutic effects.

As Paul Haun states:

> I like to think of recreation in similar terms as an important means of increasing the effectiveness of therapy. While not curative in itself, it helps create the milieu for successful treatment. . . . It combats the fears, the isolation and the resistances that threaten recovery.[7]

Edith Ball defines the term "recreation" as a pleasurable experience. "Recreation" therefore becomes the adjective which modifies or changes to some degree the term "recreation." This concept seems to confirm the implication that recreation may be seen as an end in itself or as a means to an end thereby facilitating a goal and implying the term "therapeutic."[8]

Using therapeutic recreation as a "helping process" which aims toward achieving positive changes or a restoration of needs in our clients, enables us to view the terms "therapeutic and rehabilitative" as synonymous.

As Thomas Collingwood points out:

> Therapeutic Recreation is relevant to the rehabilitation process in terms of how well, as a process, it meets clients' needs. As a service area within rehabilitation, Therapeutic Recreation has the potential to facilitate the rehabilitation of clients by meeting leisure, physical, psychological, social and vocational educational needs. How well Therapeutic Recreation meets these changes depends upon the effectiveness of programs and the effectiveness of recreation leaders to facilitate relevant client changes affecting rehabilitation outcome.[9]

Just as therapeutic recreation can be seen as one service area of recreation, it can be seen as one service area of the total rehabilitation process, offering great potential for fostering rehabilitation of the client.[10] Thus, the role of the therapeutic recreator within the long-term care facility is dependent upon how well we satisfy the needs of our client. The result achieved through therapeutic recreation as a rehabilitative tool is dependent upon the degree to which the therapeutic recreation specialist effects changes of a beneficial nature.

The very nature of recreation adds to its significance as a rehabilitative tool. Some studies have shown the therapeutic effects of recreation as helping to decrease the need for medication and even prolonging the will to live, especially among the elderly. Dr. Paul Haun feels that:

> contemporary medicine is coming to think less about disease and more about the people with the disease. The strength of the recreation movement is that it thinks about people, and in so doing goes beyond the limitations of medicine.[11]

Therapeutic recreation may be seen as a continuum. On one end of the scale may be participation in a recreation experience for purely pleasurable results, while on the other end we may wish to achieve positive changes or results, (as a therapy) specifically designed to meet our client's needs.

Recreation as an end in itself may be seen when viewing the client as a "total human being" who has been given the opportunity of chosing at will his own individualized recreation experience or leisure activity.

It is important here to briefly describe what we mean by a "total human being." The "total" person or "whole" being requires the ability to function in all areas of one's personality. The satisfaction of needs at the physical, cognitive, affective and social levels are necessary in maintaining the appropriate balance of one's personality. A problem in any one of these behavioral areas may influence the other areas, thereby affecting the total personality or the whole human being. In addition, disturbances in any area of one's personality may also affect one's behavior as a social being. Thus, an important objective of a recreation experience is to benefit or satisfy the "whole person or total human being."

Understanding how to use one's own leisure time in a meaningful, worthwhile manner is a contributing factor to successful client rehabilitation.[12] Although there is a variety of needs to be met, most recreation professionals agree that, through the ability to voluntarily and independently choose one's leisure pursuits, satisfaction of many of these needs can be met. Thus, participation in recreational experience and leisure pursuits can help people to live a better life whether living in the community or within the walls of a long-term care facility. Within the long-term care facility, the aged person who has the ability to use his leisure time in a constructive way will function more independently as a total human being, finding his place more readily within the total community of the institution.

To help foster positive changes, we can view recreation as more than an activity for a pleasurable experience. Thus, recreation also becomes a means to an end. Again, it is important to remember that the outcomes or changes desired in our clients will depend upon how well we meet their individual needs.

To satisfy the total being within the rehabilitation process, several needs may have to be met, including the physical, emotional, psychological, social and educational.

Therapeutic Recreation has been known to have great positive effects through the utilization of physical activities. These activities help maintain one's total physical being. Physical activities help keep the old youthful, especially in later years. As previously stated, the condition of one aspect of the total personality may affect other aspects. As a result, the aged person who lacks physical exercise and stimulation may also begin to feel less mentally stimulated and alive. As one grows older, the tendency to exercise decreases due to physical changes and diseases often associated with aging. Lack of interest or the availability of activities involving exercises may also be responsible for the decreased participation of the aged in such activity. Therefore, it becomes even more important to provide aged people with a program which will help satisfy their physical, medical and mental needs.

Therapeutic recreation has positive effects upon patient behavior regarding emotional and psychological problems as well. Participation in certain activities has resulted in increased self-esteem, increased self image, and a better feeling as a "total human being." In addition, every person, regardless of age requires the opportunity of "letting go," "venting," or releasing anxieties and pressures of everyday life. The elderly population, especially those living within the walls of the long-term care facility, must be given the opportunity for emotional outlet through recreation activities. Participation in activities which allow for emotional outlet and creative self expression (i.e. dramatic activities) has resulted in decreased stress, anxiety and depression.

The social and educational needs of our clients may be met through therapeutic recreation's ability to influence learning performance and the development of certain skills. Participation in certain activities require the patient to learn or acquire certain skills which were previously undeveloped. It is common for the aged person of a long-term care institution to become involved in activities he never took part in in earlier years. Participation in drama or learning how to paint becomes a new experience helping to satisfy the social and or educational needs of the client. More formal educational programs such as adult education courses should be available.

In order to participate in group activities, one must have an understanding of certain rules as well as be able to establish relationships with others in the group. Recreation activities help teach and develop skills to its participants. O'Morrow states:

> as people learn to play together, a basis is provided for helping to promote a sense of social awareness upon which the idea of brotherhood of man rests. To be an accepted group member, one must have social skills or social "know-how."[13]

Therapeutic recreation provides the elderly with the opportunity of increasing social awareness, thereby helping to facilitate a positive adjustment to institutional life.

The Therapeutic Recreation Process

At the beginning of this chapter, we asked what we meant by therapeutic recreation. We have begun to see that certain principles and techniques are utilized through a recreation experience to help satisfy the physical, psychological, emotional and social needs of the total human being or personality. The satisfaction of these needs (through therapeutic intervention) helps create positive changes within the personality of those involved. It is hoped that these changes will lead to the ultimate growth and development of the "total human being."

The utilization of these techniques and principles, therefore, becomes the "Therapeutic Recreation Process." What is important here is that there is no one concept of therapeutic recreation which becomes appropriate for everyone. Through an understanding of the basic principles of therapeutic recreation, it is the responsibility of the therapeutic recreation specialist to develop his own concept of therapeutic recreation to be utilized with the specific population with which he is involved.

The therapeutic recreation process, however, requires more than an understanding of a conceptualized group of theories, principles and techniques. Just as we discussed the "total being" as a group of physical, mental, emotional and social needs which must be satisfied, it may be stated that the therapeutic recreation process also represents a group of concepts which suggest a process as a "unified whole." Each of these concepts or phases can be separated or evaluated individually as we do with our own personality needs. Similarly, each phase or group of concepts become dependent upon each other, thereby providing us with the "total concept" of the therapeutic recreation process.

To understand each phase or concept of the therapeutic recreation process is not enough. The therapeutic recreation specialist must be able to utilize these principles through the recreation experience to bring about the positive changes and personality development we have discussed.

In her book, *Activities Therapy*, Ann Mosey explains how these principles can be used through activities therapy to help bring about specific positive changes which result in personality growth and development.

Mosey defines mental illness or psychosocial dysfunction as "the inability to meet one's needs in a manner that is satisfying to oneself and not detrimental to the need or satisfaction of others."[14]

She concurs that the inability of the client to satisfy certain gratification needs is located intrinsically within the client rather than within the environment. For example, she states that the man who is forced to live in an undesirable apartment due to his own fear of looking for a more suitable one, is thought to be in a state of psychosocial dysfunction. However, the same person who continues to live in his apartment because there are none available or affordable in a more desirable location, would not be thought of as being in a state of psychosocial dysfunction.[15]

Mosey believes that activities therapy is based on the assumption that psychosocial dysfunction is the lack of one or more of the following:[16]

the ability to plan and carry out a task and interact comfortably in a group

the ability to identify and satisfy needs and express emotions in an acceptable manner

an accurate perception of the self, the human and non-human environment and one's relationship to the environment

a value system that allows the individual to satisfy his needs without infringing on the rights of others

skill in carrying out required activities of daily living

the ability to work at a relatively satisfying job

enjoyment of avocational pursuits and recreational activities

the ability to interact comfortably in family and friendship relations

The therapeutic recreation specialist is concerned with treating the client during his present state. Although there may be considerable explanation for the behavior patterns established by people, our goal during activities therapy is to help change these behavior patterns to more positive ones during the present condition of the client. The need to explore the actual reasons for client behavior would be more appropriately dealt with through professional psychotherapy.

To help deal with and change these negative behavior patterns, we must first identify what the problems, feelings or poor behavior patterns might be. As Mosey points out, this may be accomplished through recreation activities by providing tasks the client is familiar with, which may help in identifying specific problems and improve upon their negative behavior patterns.

As director of a drama group for several years, I have witnessed such negative behavior patterns. The resident who refused to participate in the drama group unless she was the star of the show is one behavior pattern which requires attention.

After I identified this pattern, the resident realized she felt she would be unrecognized unless she were totally in the spotlight. Through the support of the group and me, the resident began to understand her problem, thereby changing her negative behavior pattern to a positive one.

This particular pattern can be seen very often with the aged person who refuses to participate in an activity unless he or she is in charge of the total program.

As mentioned previously, therapeutic recreation may influence learning and facilitate the development of new skills. The resident who refuses to participate in arts and crafts or a painting class because he feels useless as a human being due to a lack of skills is commonly seen. Participation in such a group with the aid of the therapist and his peer support will help the resident develop skills which will in turn create the feeling of increased self worth and positive self image. This skill may also lead to his feeling more independent and productive by being able to sell his painting or finished craft product. Both of these aspects of the therapeutic recreation process may be interdependent.[17] One is just as important as the other and one does not necessarily cause the other. However, a delineation of the two aspects helps the therapist define and evaluate which areas of the total therapeutic process need to be developed for each particular client.[18]

More than one area can also be worked on simultaneously. For example, the primary goal of joining the painting class was to learn or develop a new skill to help increase one's self image. At the same time, the participant may now become more independent and self sufficient by selling his product at the annual crafts fair, thus earning a small extra income. Thus, he has developed a new skill as well as helped satisfy an emotional need to feel more independent.

Within the total concept of the therapeutic recreation process, it is important to remember that when a person has a psychosocial dysfunction or when a person is ill, or impaired, only certain aspects of his personality may be limited or affected. As described in the above examples, a number of possible behavioral limitations may be present due to illness or impairment. However, there still remains many aspects of the personality which function adequately and are not effected by illness or impairment. It is the remaining unaffected areas of the personality which the therapeutic recreation specialist must work with to help facilitate positive behavioral changes. Focus upon the remaining areas unaffected by illness and disability will help prevent further deterioration or functional loss.

Avedon refers to greater functional loss or further behavioral limitations as "secondary disability."[19] As he notes, disability therefore implies the inability to deal with certain aspects of the environment resulting from physical or mental impairments. Loss of function usually results from impairment caused by disease or social conditions. Impairments caused by disease are usually irreversible and permanent. However, other disabilities caused by social conditions (i.e. social isolation of the nursing home resident) may result from neglect or merely disuse. Thus, the result of disabilities caused by such conditions may lead to decreased ability to function in any or all of the behavioral areas such as the cognitive, sensory motor or affective. Any further deterioration unrelated to the disease process has been referred to by Avedon as "secondary disabilities." What is important here, is that as Avedon concurs, "secondary disability can be prevented, delayed, limited or reversed."[20] The importance of the therapeutic recreation process becomes evident in helping to prevent further deterioration of one's behavioral limitations. It therefore becomes the specific responsibility of the therapeutic recreation specialist to help delay or reverse secondary limitation through activity therapy. Working with the healthy aspect of the personality through a well balanced, meaningful program of recreation activities, will help prevent secondary disability and will eliminate isolation or decreased social interaction in recreation activities.

One must be aware, however, that utilizing the therapeutic recreation process to bring about personality changes is not always as simple or clearcut as it may sound in our discussion. Although the therapeutic recreation process provides a milieu necessary to create positive changes, such changes do not come about naturally through the recreation experience. It becomes the responsibility of the recreation specialist to help bring about positive change through the therapeutic recreation process. This may require the activity leader to assist his client in changing certain behavior patterns, as well as reeducating him regarding his leisure needs, thereby providing for and facilitating a truly recreative experience.

The true value of the therapeutic recreation process becomes evident when the therapeutic recreation specialist intervenes, helping to move his client along the therapeutic recreation continuum. Achieving life satisfaction and the ability to function as a "total human being" within one's environment, becomes the main objective of the therapeutic recreation process. To accomplish this goal, we must understand what the problem is, develop a plan to solve it, implement the plan and finally evaluate it. Chapter Four, Developing a Well Balanced Program, has been written to help the reader accomplish this goal.

SUMMARY

Understanding therapeutic recreation, requires a knowledge base which defines the term "recreation" within a variety of contexts. The elements of this definition will help delineate the characteristics of therapeutic recreation as a process. As one specialized area within the entire field of recreation, the underlying principles and procedures of the therapeutic recreation process will help maximize the total functioning ability of its client.

Evaluation of one's physical and or psychological limitations are essential considerations in effecting changes. The therapeutic recreation specialist, therefore, becomes the catalyst in facilitating the beneficial effects of the therapeutic process. The level of assistance the client receives along the therapeutic recreation continuum will bear a direct relationship to the degree to which the client will benefit from such services.

The losses experienced by the elderly are heightened with their admission to the long-term care facility. It becomes imperative for the therapeutic recreation specialist to help open as many avenues as possible, fostering an appropriate leisure lifestyle within the walls of a new living environment.

Chapter 2

THERAPEUTIC RECREATION

Historical Implications

RECREATION AND ITS BEGINNINGS

The term "history" has been defined as "a systematic act of any set of natural phenomenon or events that shape the course of the future."[1]

If we were to open our history books and turn back the pages of time, we would certainly find a transformation of events which have helped form the recreation movement. "Recreation" and its implications have probably existed as far back as the beginning of civilization. However, the ability to define clearly what we mean by "recreation" did not exist until much later.

Historical evidence points to civilizations engaged in activities which today may be considered recreation. The use of these activities varied with each civilization and culture. Some civilizations were known to believe that illness or sickness were caused by evil spirits or demons. Many tribes used spiritual songs and dances to help ward off these evil spirits. Costumes and make-up were often part of these elaborate and dramatic rituals.

In Egypt, priests were used to help cure sick people by offering rituals to dispel the evil Gods.[2] Evidence has been found of other "recreation" activities, some carved out of slabs of stone, others in the form of cave paintings which represented recreation activities such as fishing or hunting.

The structure of society during Egyptian times resulted in recreation for the wealthy class only. Those of the peasant class devoted their time to satisfying their Egyptian ruler.

The ancient Greek civilization was instrumental to the early beginnings of the recreation movement. Their concern with satisfying their spiritual and physical needs resulted in the Greek games. These games were performed to honor their gods and were related to religious ceremonies and inspirations. Musical events and activities to satisfy intellectual needs were also initiated by such Greek philosophers as Plato.

During the time of the Protestant Reformation, leisure pursuits were viewed as negative. There was no time for play during a period which required long hours of labor. Anyone not working was seen as not contributing to the economic need of the day. Thus, the settlers of our original colonies were viewed negatively if they engaged in any recreation activities.

With the passage of time, the United States became a more industrialized nation. Society continued to change along with its needs for greater personal, physical and emotional satisfaction. As America matured, leisure pursuits or recreation activities became a more acceptable channel by which to satisfy basic human needs of pleasure and fun.

With the acceptance of "recreation" as a worthwhile way of achieving satisfaction and enjoyment, some began to see recreation as having additional benefits. Further changes during the eighteenth and nineteenth centuries which were centered around society's needs resulted in a greater concern for the care and treatment of the mentally ill population. Some institutions began implementing recreation activities for more than just diversional purposes. Certain recreation activities were now being utilized as a therapeutic intervention as their worth and therapeutic value for treatment with the mentally retarded was recognized.[3]

THE RECREATION MOVEMENT

Further changes and events continued to occur helping to form the therapeutic recreation profession. War brought about an additional set of needs for society. The American Red Cross during World War I helped provide recreation services to the wounded servicemen of hospitals and convalescent centers.[4] This was also a period of greater public awareness for recreation needs as a society at large. "The public began to realize that a well organized recreation program could accomplish much in the way of a better lifestyle for Americans."[5] World War II continued to exert the need for recreation services to military personnel. During this time the American Red Cross as well as volunteer servicemen began to find a place for themselves by implementing recreation services in hospitals throughout the country.

This became a milestone for the recreation movement. Recreation therapists or hospital recreation workers were being hired in Veterans Hospitals and military centers as well as in state facilities for the mentally retarded. With this movement came the need to organize into professional organizations.

Thus, once again historical events continued to bring change. Social concerns for the mentally retarded and wounded servicemen led to the organization of therapeutic recreation services in the early twentieth century. Beginning as volunteers through the American Red Cross and Veterans Administration hospitals, the importance of recreation services was recognized, facilitating the formal organization and public support of therapeutic recreation as a profession.

With the basis of a foundation now laid for a professional organization of therapeutic recreation, it was time to begin to develop and expand the services demanded by this new organization and movement. The postwar period, and the changes of the decades to follow provided the framework for development and expansion of therapeutic recreation services as a profession.

The period following World War II facilitated great change in the health care system of our country. Hospitals continued to expand, increasing their range of services. This resulted in the need for greater health care insurance and the ability to receive care whether one could afford it or not.[6]

With the expansion of care came an increased specialization within the medical field including psychiatric and rehabilitative services. This resulted in the need for health care workers who required education within their specialized field of care. The expansion of care and the establishment of specialization fields related to medicine helped pave the way for new types of health care facilities, including those which cared for the mentally ill, and chronically sick. In their book, *Problems, Issues and Concepts in Therapeutic Recreation*, Reynolds and O'Morrow discuss these changes which played an important role within the field of therapeutic recreation. In 1963 the Department of Health, Education and Welfare established a traineeship program in recreation for the ill and handicapped. These programs were the basis for the growth and development of specialized training in the recreation area and signified the first recognition by a federal agency of the importance of recreation services to the ill and disabled. Later legislation continued to support the value of therapeutic recreation services.[7]

The impetus of the recreation movement resulted in the establishment of professional organizations which also had an important effect upon the recreation field. In 1948 the hospital sections of the American Recreation Society was formed and was officially recognized in 1949. The American Alliance of Health, Physical Education and Recreation was formed in 1952 with a Recreation Therapy section which consisted mainly of those working in special schools whose backgrounds included recreation and physical education.[8] In 1953, the National Association of Recreation Therapists was established for those recreation workers who were employed mainly in private and public schools for the mentally ill.[9] Each of these newly formed organizations printed their own publications which reflected differences in philosophies and programs. Out of these differences grew the desire to unite in one organization to share ideas and channel communications, Thus, the Council for the Advancement of Hospital Recreation was established and this helped further common interests and concerns. More importantly, the establishment of standards for qualifications of hospital workers was incorporated through the National Voluntary Registration Program within the total recreation movement.[10]

By the 1950's the recreation movement had begun to take hold, gaining strength and expanding into several different hospital settings. However, in spite of their growth, they were still viewed by the medical field as providing service of a pleasurable nature rather than as a source of therapeutic intervention. Eventually, physicians and psychiatrists began to recognize the role and value of recreation service within the total care of the patient. Finally, the American Medical Association recognized therapeutic recreation service as an allied health field resulting from:

> recreation's contribution to the promotion of health, the prevention of
> illness or further disability, the treatment of illness, and the rehabilitation
> of persons with physical, psychological, mental or social disabilities.[11]

Paralleling the acceptance of recreation as a therapeutic intervention came an increased number of recreation curricula available in colleges and universities. Reynolds points out that the first national conference on college training of recreation leaders, conducted at the University of Minnesota in 1938, recognized "Recreation Therapy" as a specialization.[12]

The educational curriculum was further refined following conferences held regarding the role and function of the recreation specialist. Following a major conference in 1961 the term "therapeutic recreation" became the official title used to recognize recreation for the mentally ill and retarded as well as hospital recreation or recreation therapy.

As the needs of society continued to change there arose an increased awareness of the disabled population of America. As a result, therapeutic recreation expanded its service into areas other than hospital and health settings. Therapeutic recreation found its way into community areas and city based agencies as well.

The recreation movement had grown significantly by the late 1960s. Concomitant with its growth came recreation professionals and organizations which served their clients through a variety of specialized recreation areas.

The need to unify all recreation professionals regardless of the organization which provided their service, resulted in the establishment of the National Recreation and Park Association (NRPA). Under the auspicies of the NRPA other branches were established to meet the needs of specific recreation service areas. In October 1966, the National Therapeutic Recreation Society (NTRS) was established to help satisfy the needs and interests of recreation professionals involved in recreation for the ill and disabled.

The stormy, uncertain years which lead to the formation of therapeutic recreation as a profession and occupation were paralleled through the 1970's and 1980's with the need to develop a philosophy and ideology which would represent the true meaning and feeling of therapeutic recreation service. The NTRS tackled this problem unsuccessfully for several years as they focused more on the need to attain professional status and increased visibility within the area of community service. Between the 1970s and early 1980s the NTRS revised their voluntary registration program and established a new registration program based on a professional and nonprofessional level. By 1982, the NTRS had finally adopted a philosophical position statement, which was approved by its board of directors. However, the adoption of a philosophical statement does not automatically provide us with professional status. The importance of developing a philosophy and goal for therapeutic recreation will be discussed in detail in the next chapter.

SUMMARY

As one reflects upon the roads we traveled through the decades of uncertainty, it is apparent that great progress has been made within the field of therapeutic recreation. However, this progress must serve as the impetus to continue our struggles in becoming a more unified profession.

Educational curricula requires greater expansion, and certification and licensure should demand a higher level of qualification. Our voice as a professional occupation needs to be heard through our services in all areas demanded by its population.

As an occupation which has struggled to obtain professional status, we must now look into the future in hopes of achieving even greater progress for both our professional status and for the long-term care client we serve every day of our professional lives.

Chapter 3

DEVELOPING A PHILOSOPHY AND GOAL

Through the historical evolution of the recreation movement came the provision of services to the ill and disabled. Our growth as a profession has been precipitated by the changing needs of society throughout the past decades. We have provided recreation services for purely recreational purposes as well as for achieving some kind of therapeutic result. The variety of services we provide to the number of populations we serve has led to the need for a well defined philosophy and goal. The formation of therapeutic recreation as a profession and occupation has resulted in the need to develop a philosophy and ideology which would represent the true meaning and feeling of therapeutic recreation service. As Howard Danford points out, without a clear-cut philosophical ideology our program would have lacked purpose, direction and significance.

> History teaches us that no society can survive unless it has values in which the majority of its members believe deeply and that threats to that society originating from the outside are less dangerous than the slow, subtle, corrosive wearing away of faith in the ideals which first contributed to its greatness.[1]

As professionals, we must be able to share a common philosophy and set of goals which will provide a sense of unity essential to carrying out our services. The greater our values and the more we believe in them the easier it becomes to influence and inspire those who use our service.[2] The strength we obtain through the unity of our beliefs, philosophy and goals will facilitate an even greater period of professional growth. Not only must we continue to grow in the number of agencies we serve, but of equal importance is the need for a unification of beliefs to maintain the effectiveness of our service as we grow.

The need to grow through our ideological beliefs is essential to the development of our profession in areas such as certification, education, research and the techniques utilized through the therapeutic recreation process.

The decades preceding May 1982 represented periods of great controversy regarding the beliefs which were finally incorporated into the statement of philosophy adopted by the National Therapeutic Recreation Society. A knowledge and awareness regarding some of these differing positions will result in a greater understanding of the philosophy and ideology which now represents the therapeutic recreation profession as a whole.

THE GREAT DEBATES

By the late 1960s debates among recreation professionals who shared different educational backgrounds and professional training seemed to be emerging with two distinct ideological beliefs and philosophies.

One belief was that recreation was therapeutic by nature and therefore connoted that therapy was synonymous with treatment. Thus, the use of therapeutic recreation had as its goal the rehabilitation of disease or illness. As a result, some viewed themselves as recreation "therapists," while others who were considered recreation workers, dealt mainly with the recreation interest of their client.

The concomitant effects of recreation as a "therapy" were fiercely debated upon by representatives of the medical profession. Dr. Paul Haun was one who opposed the belief that recreation could be viewed as a "therapy."

> It seems both hazardous and unnecessary to me for those interested in recreation to place their figurative eggs in as gossamer a basket as "therapy;" hazardous because I know of no evidence that recreation is an effective treatment instrument and unnecessary since I am persuaded that highly relevant arguments can be advanced for providing recreational services in terms other than therapy. I am so fully persuaded of the value of recreation that I am alarmed at the possibility of its being unjustly discredited through laying claim to an effectiveness it cannot possess.[3]

Others disagreed with the position of Dr. Haun, believing, rather, that because therapy had pre-determined objectives consisting of specific goals which helped create change in the client, therapeutic recreation could be viewed as a "therapy."

The early 1970s brought a new philosophical approach which seemed to be somewhat of a compromise position between recreation for recreation's sake and recreation as a therapy.

In her article, "The Meaning of Therapeutic Recreation," Edith Ball proposed that the term "recreation" could be adapted by the use of a modifier: namely, the term "therapeutic." Thus, recreation was seen as a continuum which began as recreation for recreation's sake and continued along its continuum where it could also become therapeutic recreation.[4] Others supported this view, including the ability of therapeutic recreation to help counsel its client utilizing the educational aspects of therapeutic recreation as well.

The diversity of these debates and beliefs helped give birth to certain underlying basic principles upon which our current ideologies rest. These include the beliefs by many that:

Recreation is a specific and systematic process through which its therapeutic intervention helps create certain behavioral changes in the client.

Therapeutic recreation cannot be considered "curative" in itself.

Therapeutic recreation as a "therapeutic intervention" helps create a milieu necessary to facilitating positive behavioral changes of the recreation client.

Recreation therapists work with the remaining abilities and skills unaffected by disease or illness.

Working with the positive aspects of one's personality and physical strengths helps facilitate the growth and development of the "total being or individual."

The variety of issues and beliefs set forth by the recreation professionals of the 1960s, 1970s and 1980s culminated in a philosophical statement approved by the board of directors of the National Therapeutic Recreation Society and finally adopted by them in May, 1982. All recreation professionals should be aware of this statement and its implications upon service delivery for clients in every type of social institution. (See Appendix I for the Philosophical Position Statement of the National Therapeutic Recreation Society.)

The philosophy which underlies the growth of our field is still in its infant stage. We must strive for the continued growth of the recreation field through the advanced research, education and practice demanded by the needs of our ever-changing client population and society.

DEVELOPING A PERSONAL PHILOSOPHY AND GOAL: IMPLICATIONS OF THE LEISURE ABILITY APPROACH

The inherent principles which govern therapeutic recreation as well as our own individual beliefs and ideologies must be utilized to develop the philosophical framework necessary for the establishment and implementation of recreation programming within the long-term care facility.

The leisure ability approach developed by Gunn and Peterson and adopted by the National Therapeutic Recreation Society as the essence of its philosophical position statement has had a major impact on the delivery of recreation services. A greater understanding of its implications may provide additional ideologies and philosophies to be utilized in planning and implementing a comprehensive delivery service of recreation programming in the long-term care facility.

The changing needs of society since the Protestant Reformation has placed a much more important role on the leisure of our people. Leisure has been influenced by the values or behaviors we believe in. These beliefs and values are the result of our life's experiences. The interrelationships of our family, education, economic need, and ethnic experiences become the essence of our leisure lifestyle.

Regardless of our status in life due to physical and or psychological limitations, every person is entitled to receive equal opportunities for leisure involvement. As the leisure ability approach states: "the purpose of therapeutic recreation is to facilitate the development, maintenance, and expression of an appropriate leisure lifestyle for individuals with physical, mental, emotional or social limitations."[5] Thus, the significance of the leisure ability approach lies in its philosophy and effort at providing services which facilitate the optimal level of leisure involvement regardless of the limitations of its client. The philosophy sets the foundation for a network of services implemented through the specific areas of "therapy, leisure education and recreation participation."[6] Following an assessment of the client's specific leisure needs, the program planner will determine which area of service is required and most appropriate.

TREATMENT AND THERAPY AREA

As discussed earlier, treatment or therapy is synonymous with rehabilitation. These definitions therefore imply the process of some type of positive behavioral change fostering the maximum level of functioning of the client. Thus, the treatment component of the leisure ability approach addresses these behavioral changes within the cognitive, sensory, motor and affective behavioral arenas.

Within the long-term care facility, the treatment oriented component plays a significant role in the rehabilitation of its client. It is essential for the program planner to assess his client's needs in relation to his leisure attitudes and recreation behavioral patterns. Specifically designed programs within this area, based upon individual need, will help facilitate positive behavioral changes. These changes will lead, not only to a meaningful program of activities, but will facilitate a better overall adjustment to institutional life. The resident who is able to foster positive change will more likely function as a "total human being" in all areas of his environment.

Leisure Education Area

The leisure education area of the philosophical position statement has great implications for the program planner of the long-term care facility.

As previously stated, leisure is the free time spent enjoying leisure and recreation activities. For the elderly, most of their earlier days were spent working and rearing families. The Puritan ethic of the American agricultural society allowed little time for leisure; hence, most people were unable to develop appropriate values and leisure related attitudes. Many of these people are now the clients of the long-term care facilities or nursing homes.

It therefore becomes imperative for the program planner to provide opportunities for developing leisure skills and knowledge which will result in a greater understanding and use of leisure time for the elderly resident.

Due to the special nature of the long-term care facility population, the activity director must also teach the resident how to use his leisure skills in relation to his disability or limitation. Thus, programs will need to be developed to help change leisure attitudes and leisure awareness and interests, taking into consideration the disability areas of the resident population.

Recreation Participation

The recreation participation area plays a major role within the long-term care facility. It is to be hoped that the ability to provide the opportunity for client rehabilitation and changes in leisure attitudes will result in a meaningful program of therapeutic recreation activities which will satisfy the leisure needs of the client. Within this area, recreation activities should be developed to provide satisfaction for the total personality within the physical, cognitive, emotional and social realms. Utilization of the available modalities and techniques of therapeutic recreation should be used to provide the resident with individual choice and voluntary selection of activities.

A well planned program of activities will include activities which satisfy the intellectual, religious, social, educational, diversional and physical needs of the resident. The use of all available resources beyond those provided by the nursing home should be considered.

Whether or not the Therapeutic Recreation Service Model developed by Gunn and Peterson is used in program design, the broad principles and overall philosophy of the leisure ability approach should be considered in developing a philosophy and goal for program implementation in the long-term care facility.

THE NEED FOR A THERAPEUTIC MILIEU

The development of a philosophical position, especially in a long-term care facility, is essential to the implementation of therapeutic recreation services. Of equal importance is the milieu necessary for carrying out the goals, beliefs, and purposes inherent in the philosophy of the activities program.

As discussed, a variety of physical, psychological, emotional and social needs of the patient must be met. Each one of these needs which comprises the "total being" is equally important and dependent upon each other in maintaining a well balanced personality. Thus, in the long-term care facility, each of these needs must be met through the availability of essential services such as dietary, medical, nursing, social service and recreation. Just as the lack of any one of these services will affect the total being of the patient, it is the combination of all of these essential services which helps create the milieu or environment necessary for the patients to live a meaningful life. Because each discipline provides an essential service to the "total well being" of the resident, no one department can substitute services for the other. It therefore becomes the responsibility of the administrator to create a milieu which facilitates the significance of a well balanced activities program. Through the tone and therapeutic environment created by the administrator, staff members of every department must support the value of the activities program. As Phyllis Foster writes:

> Long-term care makes it necessary to meet the needs of individuals that may extend from those who have lost all touch with the real world, to those able to make their own decisions and proceed with establishing a new lifestyle. It is vital to the resident that everyone involved with him, from his family to his physician, support and accept the value of the activities program as necessary to his total health care.[7]

SUMMARY

Developing a personal philosophy and goal are essential to the adequate delivery of therapeutic recreation services. The underlying principles of the leisure ability approach offered by Gunn and Peterson in the philosophy position statement of the National Therapeutic Recreation Society, provide a basis for which ideologies and philosophies can be expanded.

Just as the development of a philosophical statement for the activities program is essential to its implementation, so is the support and acceptance of the administration in promoting the value of the activities program for the total well being of its patient population. Administrative support should include the reinforcement of the program's philosophy which reflects the belief, goals and attitudes of the long-term care facility.

Chapter 4

DEVELOPING A WELL BALANCED PROGRAM

The building of a sound delivery system of therapeutic recreation service in some ways parallels the construction of a well designed edifice. It is just as easy to slap together the bricks of a building as it is for a recreation director to provide some type of a recreation program for his clients.

However, one of the most important jobs of designing a well balanced program is the need to establish an overall blue print which offers direction in determining the plans, philosophy and goals of the program.

Elliot Avedon suggests that recreation programming was not always done on a systematic basis.

> Most recreation program planning in the past has been based upon lists of principles. These lists, while promulgating a range of positive social values, are nonsystematic and do not lend themselves to specific procedures that result in definitive and measurable outcomes.[1]

Avedon found that several recreation texts promulgated certain guidelines which, although they offer appropriate principles, do not lend themselves to a systematized approach to program planning. These guidelines included the phrase "program should" or "program must" with the following intentions:[2]

be developed to meet important needs

be planned realistically with regard to participants

be efficient

consider existing services and potential resources

have diversity and balance

involve challenge

ensure maximum participation

possess adequate financial support

include thoughtful evaluations

demonstrate imaginative use of resources

use qualified leadership and supervision

Thus, program planning and design encompasses more than the implementation of a variety of activities based upon well intended principles. Program planning requires a systematized goal oriented approach built upon the following:

A basic understanding of what we mean by recreation

A thorough knowledge of the techniques, principles and procedures of therapeutic recreation as a process

The development of an appropriate goal and philosophy based upon the needs of the client and its agency

Assessment of client needs in all relevant areas of functioning

Analysis, adaptation and selection of appropriate activities as they relate to the resident's disabilities

Ongoing evaluation of program achievement, staff and facilities

METHODS OF PROGRAM PLANNING

A variety of approaches to program planning appears throughout the literature. Howard Danford identifies some of these approaches and the problems inherent in them.[3]

The Traditional Approach

This method relies upon what the program has been for the past several years. Due to the success of the program in the past, there seems to be little need to change. However, this approach does not allow for changes in client population, personnel changes and most important, advances in the recreation field due to improvements in new methods and techniques.

The Current Practices Approach

This approach relies upon what others are doing. Here, the activity director utilizes the successful elements of other activity programs. However, the success of one program does not ensure the success of another.

The elements of an activity program in one setting may not be successful in another.

The Expressed Desires Approach

This method focuses on the interests of the participants in the program. Questionnaires or interviews are used to evaluate which activities in which the clients wish to participate. The problem with this method is that the program is based on the range and scope of interests of the client, which may be limited due to his own leisure awareness or recreation experience. In addition, the program planner is not given the opportunity of introducing new programming or recreation experiences.

The Authoritarian Approach

With this approach, the activity staff makes all the decisions regarding the activities program. The obvious weakness of this approach lies in the fact that the activities staff is left to make all decisions for the recreation needs and interests of its client population independently.

These approaches need to be looked at with caution. However, as Danford notes, it does not mean there can be no good in any of these methods. For example, one cannot blindly utilize the elements of another program as is done with the "current practices approach." However, if one looks carefully, there may be certain elements that can be used in another program. Thus, a combination of ingredients from one or all of the methods discussed may be helpful in designing a well balanced program.

ESSENTIAL ELEMENTS OF PROGRAM DESIGN

Certain factors must be considered regardless of the method or approach utilized to design a therapeutic recreation program. These elements are essential ingredients common to the design of *any* program and warrant further examination. The following criteria need to be investigated as part of the design of a well balanced program for delivery of therapeutic recreation services.

The author will examine these factors as they relate specifically to the design of therapeutic recreation programming in the long-term care facility. It would benefit the reader to address this information to the specific type of long-term care facility he may be involved in.

Assessing the Nature of the Client

Before we can begin to design a recreation program we need to know who we are designing the program for. Are we planning a program for the elderly population of a nursing home or for the disturbed person of a mental facility? It is obvious that the needs of these differing populations will require a variety of interventions and techniques.

Socio-Economic background. The socio-economic status will certainly be a determinent factor in planning for recreation programming. Certain recreation and leisure pursuits may have been precluded by the economic status of the participant. Extended vacations, cruises or travel are certainly limited to those who can afford such leisure pursuits. The opportunity to experience cultural events such as broadway plays, concerts, opera and theatrical events are certainly limited by one's economic status. Similarly, the opportunity to participate in spectator sports (baseball games, football, etc.) may also be economically prohibitive to some. Thus, the lack of exposure to such events may limit the leisure interests of those whose socio-economic backgrounds prohibit participation in this type of recreation experience.

James Murphy indicates that the first national recreation survey in Britain showed that:

> the higher the income level, occupational class and educational status of contacts, the greater the number of pursuits they mentioned for their weekend before interview and the greater the importance of the "active" compared with the "passive" recreations. In short, those with the highest socio-economic status not only do more things, but do more active things.[4]

The leisure lifestyle of the resident will therefore be based in part, upon the varying degree of exposure to activities according to socio-economic status. Hence, it becomes important to examine the socio-economic backgrounds of those in the long-term care facility to help determine the differences in activity interests and the level of involvement in such leisure experiences.

Educational background. The educational background of the long term care participant may also affect participation in recreation programming. Studies have indicated that the higher the level of education, the greater the scope of recreational interests. Thus, those with less formal education may be more limited in their recreational interests.

Occupational background. The level of education one reaches may directly affect the type of occupation he chooses for his career. The occupational background of the participant will therefore affect his choice of recreation and leisure pursuits. For example, a participant who was a professional person will probably have different leisure pursuits than someone who may have held a blue collar job. Murphy indicates that certain

American studies link occupation with leisure interests. A study by Joel Gerstl suggests, "college professors spent less time with their children and around the home and less time on sport and nonprofessional organizations than did either admen or dentists.[5]

Examining the socio-economic, educational and occupational status becomes an important determinant in program planning. The number or percentage of participants with differing backgrounds in each of these areas needs to be examined. The following table may help the therapeutic recreation specialist to distinguish which levels of each area need to be investigated.

Ethnic and religious background. The ethnic and religious background of the client's population plays an essential role in program planning. The customs and traditions of ethnic groups will certainly affect their choice of activities.

Musical programs of nursing homes may depend upon the ethnic background of its client population. For example, residents of a predominantly Jewish nursing home may enjoy participating in musicals which offer Jewish or Israeli music. The importance of refreshments at activities as well as the type of refreshment served may also be dependent upon the ethnic group being served.

Ethnic backgrounds may also determine which holidays will be observed or not observed in certain facilities, as well as how the holidays will be observed.

Religious backgrounds and practices also affect participation in activ-

Table 4-1: Background Assessment of Client

Socio-economic Status:	Educational Status:	Occupational Status:
% in facility	% in facility	% in facility
Lower class	Elementary	Blue Collar
Upper-lower	school	
	(Grades 1–6)	White Collar
Lower-middle		
Upper-middle	Middle	Professional
	school	
Lower-upper	(Grades 7–9)	
Upper class		
	High school	
	(Grades 9–12)	
	College	
	Post Graduate	
	Vocational	

ities. Certain religions may determine when activities may or may not be held. Certain nursing homes may require that no recreation activities be held on the Sabbath since this day is reserved for prayers and rest. Religious practices of other denominations may require prayers or church services on a daily basis.

Thus, the number or percentage of similar ethnic or religious backgrounds in any particular setting will certainly help determine how to plan programs for this particular population.

Age and age-related factors. What is the average age of the client? What is the age range of the client population?   The age of those in long-term care facilities or nursing homes will be a crucial factor to consider. However, it is important to remember that chronological age does not necessarily reflect the ability or performance level of the client at hand. Deterioration or decline in the elderly may vary. Observations of the elderly in recreation activities indicate that physical and/or mental deterioration occurs at different stages of life, not necessarily related to one's chronological age. Thus, one's ability or limitation must be based upon the level of physical, psychological or social growth or deterioration rather than chronological age. As observed through recreation activities, an older person may exhibit increased confusion while others may be declining physically. Therefore, although activity interests vary with age, it is not the chronological age which determines the type of activity to plan for, but the development or decline of the resident's abilities in the sensory motor, affective or cognitive areas.[6]

Gender. How many clients are being served by your program? How many males are there in the facility? How many females are there in the facility? Traditionally, activity directors and program planners experience some difficulty in satisfying the needs of male participants. Some have observed that biological and cultural factors may affect the participation pattern of males and females. Society has affixed certain "cultural expectations" upon each gender, and it would seem that these expectations limit or affect the participation in activities for the male population more than for the females in long-term care settings. The economic need to work and support a family limited their past participation in recreation activities. Males were "expected" to work. Their leisure experiences were limited to playing cards or watching the popular sport of the day. On the other hand, the woman's role created a broader range of recreation or leisure interests, although they, too, had their own "expected" roles. Many women, however, included as their leisure the need to sew, knit, cook or garden. Thus, these types of activities seem to invite wider scheduling.

It should be noted that biological differences may also have affected recreation participation. The male often requires activities which demand greater physical dexterity. Men's desire for sports, exercise or crafts such as woodworking or metalworking suggests differences in the recreation needs of the genders. Thus, to foster appropriate program planning, it is important to consider the different needs of the two sexes.

Disabilities.   An understanding of the client's disabilities is crucial to the development of program planning. A later chapter will discuss Activity Analysis, which will allow us to break down the inherent elements of each activity, fostering an awareness of the skills necessary for participation in that activity. Although activity analysis may be done independently of client needs, the process utilized has many implications for therapeutic recreation programming. Activity analysis is an essential step toward enabling the adaptation or modification of activities for clients with functional disabilities. In short, once an activity is analyzed for essential components, it may be modified to meet the needs of the client, dependent upon their disability. Thus, an assessment of the client's disabilities and their severity in all relevant areas is necessary.

Program planning is dependent upon the ability of the client to participate in recreation activities. The abilities and skills required for participation may be limited by disorders in any of the three behavioral arenas. It is essential to understand how these disabilities affect our client so we can avoid asking them to use the skills or abilities which may be impaired. Understanding the implications of disabilities in each behavioral area may affect program planning. The following table will help delineate disabilities affecting program planning.

Table 4-2: Behavioral Disabilities Affecting Program Planning

Behavioral Area:	*Disabilities Affecting Participation*
Sensory-Motor (Body movements—motor skills)	Poor ambulation Poor gait Poor bodily movements and strength Poor vision Poor hearing
Cognitive (Intellectual functioning)	Inability to recognize information Inability to store and retrieve information Inability to make appropriate judgements Inability to maintain attention span
Affective Area (Emotions, feelings)	Depression Apathy Anxiety Anger Fear Frustration Agitation

Secondary disabilities. Disability or impairment may cause behavioral limitations in any of the areas noted above. To help prevent further limitations or increased functional loss, the therapeutic recreation specialist works with the unaffected part of the personality or behavioral arena. Thus, secondary disability is referred to as a disability resulting from a primary condition which may lead to even greater deterioration or loss for the resident. This loss will create a further decline in his ability to function within the behavioral areas discussed. Great emphasis must be placed upon the importance of secondary disability, as this can be reversed or prevented. For example, an elderly resident whose primary condition is hearing loss, may tend to isolate himself, resulting in greater functional loss. Thus, an awareness of the types of disabilities present in the client population is crucial to the program planner. As Avedon explains:

> Secondary disability need not be a permanent condition, for the residual factors that cause it can be reversed, prevented, or delayed if proper services are made available. When this is not done, there is rapid withdrawal from social interaction and involvement in activities of a social nature. When this happens, one has become handicapped.[7]

Population trends. Program planning demands attention to the population trends occurring within a given facility.

Previous years brought the admission of more alert, able-bodied elderly to nursing home facilities. However, the increasing number of community outreach services has resulted in a dramatic rise of elderly who are able to live with assistance in their homes for a longer period of time. By the time these people seek admission to a nursing home, they are sicker, more frail and less independent than those of past decades. Program planning therefore requires careful attention to the changing needs of those admitted to the long-term care facility.

Leisure lifestyle. In addition to assessing client needs, information related to leisure interests, attitudes and activity preferences is required. Thus, the leisure lifestyle of the population being served becomes an important factor to consider. Questions such as the following need to be asked:

> What was the leisure lifestyle of the client previous to admission to the nursing home?
>
> What was the client's level of participation in community events and social events?
>
> What was the client's level of participation in social organizations?
>
> Is the client aware of the need to plan for leisure interests?
>
> What are the values, attitudes and behaviors in relation to leisure?

Questions such as these can be asked through group interventions or individualized preference questionnaires. Evaluating and re-evaluating activity preferences and attitudes toward leisure is an important element not only in program planning, but in maintaining the interests of those already participating in the activities program.

Every client admitted to a long-term care facility requires an evaluation of his leisure needs and interests, which will result in an individualized treatment plan. The process of initial interviewing is essential to program planning and will be discussed in greater detail in Chapter Ten, "The Paperwork Dilemma."

Assessing the Agency

In addition to analysis of the client population, several factors must be analyzed in relation to the agency one is involved in.

As previously stated, developing a well balanced program is dependent upon its reason for existence and its purpose and goals. Just as important for the program planner is an understanding of the reason for being and overall goals and objectives of the agency itself. Each agency will have its own statement of purpose and goals which will determine the types of services offered. An understanding of the specific goals of the entire agency is essential to the development of a therapeutic recreation program.

History. Just as the background or history of the client is important, so is the history of the facility. An understanding of who, why and where the organization or agency began may be helpful in explaining why certain services are carried out by the facility. Certain agencies may be more progressive than others, taking on new challenges and expanding services whenever possible. On the other hand, there are agencies whose services may be dictated by years of tradition which may not be appropriate to the changes and trends of its client population. These differences may be directly related to the values or beliefs of the founders or organizers of the facility.

Organizational structure. Understanding the organizational structure of the long-term care facility is important and necessary for the program planner. An awareness of the facility's organizational structure will foster smoother inter-departmental communication and cooperation. Support and communication between the nursing and activity department, for example, will facilitate help in transporting residents to activities. No department operates in a vacuum. Each department is dependent upon others for certain needs, which results in the success of the total program.

Regulatory standards. The type and extent of services provided by long-term care facilities are in part determined by the agencies which regulate support and accredit them. Of equal importance is an understanding of these regulations and standards which affect the delivery of therapeutic recreation services. Such regulatory bodies may include the Joint Commission on Accreditation of Hospitals and the State Department of Health.

Federal, state or local mandates may also affect program requirements. In New York, the state hospital code sets specific standards and regulations which have a direct impact upon therapeutic recreation programming. A thorough knowledge and clear understanding of the state code requirements are essential to the program planner. These standards may include:

> the number of staff required
>
> the qualifications of staff
>
> the documentation of treatment plans

A review of the state code and its implications upon therapeutic recreation programming will be discussed in greater detail in Chapter Ten, "The Paperwork Dilemma."

Agency Resources

A well balanced program will also depend upon the availability of potential resources both within the facility and outside of it. An analysis of these potential resources is a necessary step for the program planner.

Staff numbers. As previously mentioned, the state code in many instances mandates the number of staff required. Certain states require activity departments to provide a specific number of staff hours for recreation activities. A careful look at the number of available staff is therefore important. A creative program planner will use the state code as a means of support if his facility lacks the appropriate number of activity staff members.

Staff qualifications. State codes may also require certain educational and professional degrees, especially for activity directors. The program planner should be familiar with these requirements. It is obvious that we all aim for the highest possible quality of activity staff.

We also need to examine the skills and abilities of the activity staff. Program content will obviously help determine which skills and abilities will be required of the activity staff.

Auxiliary staff. A creative program planner will look beyond the doors of the activities department for potential resources. The auxiliary staff (nurses aides and orderlies) may be one of the most valuable resources of the non-therapeutic recreation staff. Facilities whose goals are the total care of the patient population, will allow and encourage the help and support of the auxiliary staff in activities programs. The provision of "hands on" care is carried out by the auxiliary staff members, who probably know the patients better than anyone else in the facility. This same staff is often present in the lounge areas during activity programs. Its skills and abilities should be utilized to augment the activities program.

At The Jewish Home and Hospital for Aged, Bronx, New York, a new and exciting program has recently been instituted. This program, which is known as the Personalized Care Model (PCM), has developed a new approach to the *total* care of the patient population of its facility. An integral part of this program is the responsibility of the auxiliary staff in carrying out the total care of their assigned cluster of patients which also consists of direct involvement with the activities department.

The use of adaptive activities is one area in the total program of PCM. Through the holistic approach of the Personalized Care Model, adaptive activities becomes an umbrella under which a diversified program of therapeutic recreation activities evolve.

With the utilization of these activities, the recreation leader and the primary helper (nurses aide and orderly) provide the unique opportunity of expanding the horizon and adding a new dimension to the living environment of the institutionalized aged resident.

The combination of adaptive activities and the treatment modalities of therapeutic recreation facilitate a continuity of care, resulting in the extension of the resident's lifestyle.

Thus, the primary helper becomes an added resource through which the principles and procedures of therapeutic recreation are utilized to achieve a meaningful and worthwhile program of activities.

The development of the PCM model (by Clara and Judith Nicholson) has great implications and value for the activities program. Therefore, an overview of the entire PCM program is found in Appendix II.

Patient families.   Another potential resource are patient families. Often, family members are seen in a negative manner, having little to offer in the care of their parents, sibling or relatives. However, the use of the Friends and Relatives Association has begun to bring about positive changes. Families are being educated regarding the problems, concerns and issues that affect the daily lives of their institutionalized relatives. In many cases committees are established to work with staff members in trying to solve problems.

The increased involvement and education of families has resulted in a greater understanding of the problems faced by administrators and staff in general of long-term care facilities. Changing attitudes and greater involvement of family members are becoming an additional positive resource for the program planner. Some nursing homes work closely with family members who volunteer at holiday parties and special events throughout the year.

Volunteers. The use of volunteers in activity programs cannot be ov-eremphasized. Some facilities have a separate volunteer department while others require the activity director to act as volunteer coordinator as well. Due to the significant role of the volunteer in activity programming, a separate chapter will be devoted to this area.

Space and facilities. An analysis of available space and facilities is crucial to a well balanced program. The following questions may help in examining the appropriate facilities.

Are there terrace and/or garden areas for outdoor activities and events?

Are there adequate numbers of large and/or small activity rooms?

Are there provisions for religious service areas?

Is there a resident library?

Is there an arts and crafts room?

Are these areas easily accessible to ambulatory and non-ambulatory residents?

Are there adequate elevators and or ramps?

Is the activity office in an area easily accessible to residents?

Are there other areas in the facility which can be used by the activity department such as floor lounges or dining rooms?

Budget. The following require careful investigation.

What is the amount of the current and available budget?

Is the budget adequate for a well balanced program? (The state code may require a minimum amount to be spent on each client regarding activity supplies. The program planner should be familiar with the code.)

Who develops the budget? Is the activity director involved in preparing and developing an appropriate budget?

Are there any other sources of income available for the budget such as fund raising, private contributions, etc.?

Supplies and Equipment. A well balanced program obviously requires appropriate equipment and adequate supplies. The following questions need to be asked by the program planner:

What equipment is available to the activity program?

Piano(s)

Cassette recorder(s)

Stereo(s)

Caliphone(s)

Movie projector(s)

Slide projector(s)

Portable movie screen(s)

VCR equipment

Microphone(s)

Portable microphone(s)

Kiln(s)

Rug loom(s)

Camera(s)

What supplies are available?

Arts and crafts materials: wool, yarn, paints, construction paper, glue, etc.

Talking book machines

Large-print books and magazines

Community Resources

An important goal of the therapeutic recreation program in the long-term care facility should be to maintain whenever possible, the prior lifestyle of its client population. This can be achieved by maintaining ties with the facility and its surrounding community. The following areas may be investigated as possible community resources.

The local church or temple may provide:

Rabbinical services or a visiting clergy

Holiday programs with the children of its parish or religious school

The neighborhood schools may provide:

Holiday programs

Intergenerational programs

Escort services of students to local shopping areas

Volunteer services within the facility

Other community resources include:

Museums	Zoos	Botanical gardens
Movies	Shopping centers	
Parks	Libraries	Sports complexes

The mayor's or local politician's office may provide information regarding:

political organizations

information regarding social action

local concerts

special senior citizen programs

A local map and guide of the surrounding community should be provided to the client population. This should include:

a street map of community areas

transportation services in the neighborhood

names of local stores and restaurants

Some clients do return to their community to live. With this in mind, an awareness of the surrounding community and its available resources will facilitate an easy transition for those who return to the community.

Other Areas for Consideration

Facility location. The location of the facility will undoubtedly affect the activity program. Facilities located in or around the city will probably be closer to public transportation and community resources such as museums, parks, shopping centers, etc. Entertainers and volunteers will also be easier to obtain. Relatives will probably visit more often due to availability of public transportation or their proximity to major roads. Facilities in the city area may also be able to share resources with neighboring institutions or nursing homes. Changing city neighborhoods make it difficult or unsafe at times to walk in the community. Outdoor areas are therefore necessary.

Those facilities located out of the city limits will be limited in resources due to their lack of accessibility. These places will need to depend more on their own vehicles for transportation and outings. Volunteers and entertainers will also be more difficult to obtain. However, outdoor areas are usually more abundant or accessible in surburban facilities.

Scheduling. Admission to the long-term care facility connotes loss of freedom and individuality in many areas. The elderly resident of a nursing home becomes the victim of the social structure and organizational patterns of the institution. Individuality and independence become difficult to achieve as the life of a nursing home resident becomes divided. Dietary feeds the resident, nursing medicates him and housekeeping cleans his room. All of these services are provided at certain times, on specific days and in specific places throughout the home. Thus, adjustment to the home requires the establishment of certain patterns in the usage of time. Once the daily basic needs of the residents are met, they will be left with a period of unrestricted time. It is this unrestricted time that allows for participation in recreation activities.

Unrestricted time may vary for each resident. Therefore, program planning becomes even more difficult. Although activities may need to be scheduled when patients can attend, certain activities may not be successful during certain times of the day.[8] For example, a birthday party at which refreshments are served would probably not be well attended in the morning hours even if the patients had the time to attend.

Living within the walls of an institutional setting places a special significance upon the usage of free time. Residents are often forced to celebrate holidays and special events within the confines of the facility and often at the time the activities staff is available to work. It therefore becomes even more significant to plan programs and holiday celebrations on the day they occur. Previous to admission, residents may have spent their evenings and weekends pursuing leisure interests and activities as they saw fit. Many of these opportunities are limited within the institutional setting.

The program planner must be aware of a variety of scheduling patterns including:

holidays throughout the year

seasonal activities and special events

weekend activities

theme activities (monthly)

daily time patterns of clients

Thus, scheduling of activities and the use of free time becomes an important factor in program planning.

SUMMARY

The program planner must be acutely aware of a variety of important factors.

A logical method or approach must be considered, dependent upon the needs of the population being served. Certain elements of program design are necessary. A thorough assessment of the client and his background and disabilities, as well as the agency and its community resources is essential to the initial program planning process. The combination of all of these factors will help provide the necessary ingredients of a well balanced program.

Just as important as establishing a solid foundation for the development of a well balanced program is the selection of appropriate activities, which will be discussed in the next chapter.

Chapter 5

SELECTING APPROPRIATE ACTIVITIES

Activity Analysis

A crucial step in developing a well balanced program is the selection of appropriate activities for the therapeutic recreation program. In program selection it is important for the planner to choose activities which will help achieve resident needs as well as the goals of the overall program. One method of selecting appropriately is through activity analysis.

Activity analysis is a process which allows us to dissect the elements of an activity into its individual parts. An analysis of each individual element provides the program planner with a greater understanding of how the activity may help its client achieve successful participation. Examining the individual elements helps the program planner determine which skills and abilities are required for participation in activities. This further enables the program planner to modify or adapt appropriate activities which will allow for participation of the patient or client.

Activity analysis should not be confused with task analysis. Task analysis is a method used for articulating a step-by-step approach for teaching activity skills to the impaired patient. On the other hand, activity analysis allows for adaptation of the activity itself in facilitating patient participation.

Skills and Abilities for Activity Participation

Successful participation in any activity requires the ability to function in the physical, cognitive and affective behavioral arenas. Most activities will require skills and abilities in each of the three arenas in order to achieve a successful level of participation.[1] For example, a bowling game requires the physical ability of holding and throwing the ball as well as seeing where to throw it. The patient, however, requires the cognitive ability to think and plan where the ball should be thrown to best hit the pins. Affectively, bowling often causes feelings of excitement when all the pins are knocked down or frustration at missing the pins.

Skills and abilities may be impaired in all three behavioral arenas. Although an impairment in one arena may affect ones personality or participatory skills in the other two behavioral arenas, it is common to find that the major disorder usually occurs in one particular arena.[2]

In a previous chapter, we discussed the importance of working with the remaining abilities and positive aspects of the patients personality. Thus, it becomes crucial to the program planner to understand when a disorder results in a disability or impairment, so the client does not have to use this particular skill or ability.

Physical Arena (Sensory-Motor)

The physical arena makes it necessary to analyze each activity to determine which body movements are needed to carry out the activity. Analysis of these movements would include how the body would need to move as well which parts of the body would be utilized. Such an analysis may consider the entire musculoskeletal activity: balance, coordination, strength and the use of the five senses. For example, planning a bowling program will require analysis as outlined in the following table.

In addition to physical limitations due to sensory motor impairments, the program planner must consider the inability to participate due to certain

Table 5-1: Physical Analysis of Bowling Activity

Required Ability	Required Physical Movement
Ability to hold ball (Hand strength)	Spread fingers on hand. Place fingers into holes of bowling ball.
Eye-hand coordination (Sight)	Eyes must focus on bowling pins while arm is moving into position to lift and deliver ball.
Ability to release ball	Movement of arm to a lowered position. Pushing motion of arm. Release of ball from finger position.
Follow through	Continued movement of arm in an upward position.
Coordination of arm movement and body movement to be able to release ball at beginning of alley.*	Walking motion: one foot to move in front of the other.

*For wheelchair participants, coordination of throwing the ball and walking will not be necessary.

illnesses or disease processes. For example, patients with heart conditions, asthma, or respiratory conditions may be advised not to participate in certain activities, thereby limiting him to certain physical movements. Thus, analysis of the physical requirements of activities enables the program planner to select and adapt activities appropriate to his particular population.

Cognitive Arena

The cognitive arena has a major influence upon activity participation, affecting the intellectual functioning of the client. An impairment in this arena will have serious implications for program planning.

Intellectual functioning is more than just accepting and understanding information. As the literature points out:

> Mature and efficient cognitive processes permit the selection for attention of particular stimuli or features of stimuli to the exclusion of others, the division or distribution of attention across a stimulus field and the flexibility with respect to the focus, locus and maintenance of attention over time.[3]

Hence, the cognitive arena allows for an individual to focus upon and distinguish certain informational stimuli which may then be retrieved or stored. As a result, memory may also be affected by the cognitive arena. Both the ability to make certain judgements and evaluate certain situations are influenced by the cognitive arena. The attention span for activity participation may also be affected. In addition, the intellectual functioning allows us to interpret specific forms of communication including symbols other than the written language.

The level of participation in activities will depend greatly upon the presence of impairment in the cognitive arena. The program planner must therefore be aware of how this impairment will affect the skills or abilities of its client in activity participation.

Understanding the goal of an activity is essential for participation. A patient who does not understand what to do or why he is doing something may indulge in inappropriate behavior and be unable to participate in the activity. A resident who does not know what to do with a paint brush or paint may try to eat it. Thus, an understanding of the purpose of the activity is essential for successful participation. The program planner must consider how much the client is able to understand with regard to the intent of the program.

Understanding the rules of an activity is also essential. Cognitive impairment may make it difficult to understand the rules of an activity or game. The program planner must adapt or modify such rules based upon the cognitive ability of the client. For example, the complicated rules of a bowling game may be simplified by giving each participant ten points for knocking down all the pins.

The ability to remember must also be considered in program planning. A patient may understand the goal or rules of an activity at a particular moment. However, if his memory retention is impaired he will forget the rules a few moments later. Thus, the amount of memory as well as the amount of retention of the patient need to be considered for activity participation.

The patient's understanding of how to play a game or participate in an activity must also be considered by the program planner. Impairment in this cognitive area may limit one's ability to participate in a particular activity. It is one thing to understand the rules of a checker game but quite another to be able to use the appropriate cognitive skills in moving the pieces.

Attention span must also be considered by the program planner. Participation in a checker or bingo game may require too great an attention span for some. However, participation in a social hour or musical program may require less concentration and attention.

The ability of the patient to read and write must also be considered. Activities which require such skills must be carefully considered to ensure successful participation of the client being served.

Analysis of the cognitive arena provides the program planner with an understanding of certain behavioral limitations which affect the ability to participate in activities. This understanding is necessary in modifying or adapting activity elements to help ensure successful participation by the client.

A further understanding of the origins of the behavioral problems will ensure even greater success in adapting activity elements for the impaired person. One needs to be cautioned, however, not to change the elements discussed so that they alter the nature of the activity. It is important to distinguish between those behavioral problems which result from direct damage or deterioration to the brain and those which may result from social problems. It is important to determine if a resident is unable to communicate because of a stroke or depression or social isolation.

Thus, a thorough understanding of the cognitive arena is essential to developing a well balanced program.

Affective Arena

Just as there may be impairments in the physical and cognitive arenas, impairments in the affective arenas must also be considered.

Evaluating affective behaviors or emotional feelings are sometimes more difficult since they are not so concrete or obvious as physical problems or behavioral impairments may be.

Just as a recreation experience for one may not be a recreation experience for another, the emotions or feelings caused by a specific activity may be different for everyone participating in it. Thus, a careful look at this arena is important. The implications of emotions or feelings in activity planning is significant.

It should be noted that emotional responses may occur as a *result* of activity participation or may *prevent* participation in activities.

In the affective arena, the program planner needs to be aware of certain feelings or emotions which seem to dominate a patient's behavior, thereby preventing and/or impairing participation in activities. For example, every human has some degree of fear. However, a resident who refuses to participate because he is frightened of leaving his room, frightened of being with others or afraid of failing at a specific task, may be said to have an impairment in the affective arena. Thus, a resident whose behavior is dominated by a particular feeling or emotion will experience an impairment in this area.

The program planner must also be aware of the fact that certain emotions may result from participating in an activity. These emotions are different for every participant. The following table lists certain emotions which will provide the program planner with a better understanding of possible reactions resulting from participation or may offer clues to why the patient refuses to participate in certain activities. Thus, an understanding of the affective arena is critical to the program planning process.

SOCIAL INTERACTIONS: INTERACTIVE PROCESSES

The combination of physical and cognitive abilities and the emotional response of the client are important factors in activity participation. The variety of skills and abilities necessary for participation also demand interaction on different levels. An understanding of the level of social interaction necessary for successful participation is crucial to the program planner in selecting activities for his program. Certain patients are unable to relate to others on an individual basis. The inability to relate to others will certainly prevent that person from interacting successfully as part of a group or team or in a recreation situation.

Elliot Avedon has identified eight interactive processes that influence one's behavior while engaged in this process. Avedon indicates that the inability to master one level will prevent the person from achieving success in the next level of interaction. It is important to identify each interactive process.[4] An understanding of these patterns will help the program planner develop appropriate therapeutic goals and social skills for the resident.

Table 5-2: Emotions Affecting Activity Participation

Emotion:	Implication for Activity Participation:
Fear	May prevent participation in activity due to fear of failure. "I'm too old to participate." "I can't do anything anymore."
Agitation	May result from inability to carry out a certain task. Too many obstacles may prevent client from achieving successful participation. May also prevent participation. Symptoms may include: pacing, restlessness, aggressive behavior.
Anxiety	May result in a variety of symptoms: tension, irritability. May also result from a pleasurable activity, causing increased stimulation and awareness, i.e. participation in a play may cause anxiety.
Apathy	A feeling of indifference. Often leads to refusal to participate. May be the result of poor leisure attitudes. "I don't feel like doing anything."
Joy or Pleasure	Result of participation in a pleasurable experience or activity. The patient may have successfully completed a recreation project or may have won at a particular activity.

Intra-Individual

Action taking place within the mind of a person or action involving the mind and a part of the body, but requiring no contact with another person or external object.

i.e.: daydreaming.

This type of interaction is rarely used in therapeutic recreation programming as a structured program. However, residents do often daydream.

Extra-Individual

Action directed by a person toward an object in the environment, requiring no contact with another person.

i.e. reading, doing crossword puzzles, viewing television.

Most recreation activities require greater social skills and interaction than extra-individual activities. These types of activities, however, are important to those who enjoy being alone.

Aggregate

Action directed by a person toward an object in the environment while in the company of other persons who are also directing action toward objects in the environment. Action is not directed toward one another, and no interaction between participants is required or necessary.

i.e. bingo game, movies

Although no action is required among the group members, this type of activity serves as a starting point for developing social skills for activities which require a greater level of social interaction.

Inter-Individual

> Action of a competitive nature directed by one person toward another. The first of the true dyadic relationships.
>
> i.e. chess, checkers

Because this is an action of a competitive nature, the participant must be prepared to win or lose. Depending upon the activity, a variety of levels of interaction will be necessary. Some activities require no verbal exchange (checkers) whereas others may require greater interaction.

Unilateral

> Action of a competitive nature among three or more persons, one of whom is an antagonist or *IT*. Interaction is in simultaneous competitive dyadic relationships.
>
> i.e. exercise group.

These types of activities require greater interaction plus recognition of a leader. Most of the interaction occurs between the participant and the leader rather than among the individual members of the group.

Multilateral

> Action of a competitive nature among three or more persons, with no one person as an antagonist.
>
> i.e. card games, board games.

These types of activities require interaction among all of the group members and require that each person make individual choices or decisions.

Intra-Group

> Action of a *cooperative* nature by two or more persons intent upon reaching a mutual goal. Action requires positive verbal and nonverbal interaction. This is a true group structure. It requires the interactive process known as *cohesion*, i.e. when people in the group can resolve conflict through compromise, thus enabling the group to develop and express positive feelings for one another. The opposite process is *anomie*, i.e. when people in the group cannot resolve conflict and cannot con-

tinue the activity; anomie is the inability of the participants to "give and take" and to get along with another by arriving at a compromise.

It is essential for the participant to be able to function in a group situation. The development of social skills for successful participation in group activities is crucial. In addition to functioning in recreation activities, the resident who maintains adequate social skills will also be able to function as a total human being within the total environment of the institutional setting.

Inter-Group

Action of a competitive nature between two or more intra-groups. Participants who have been unable to relate or who lack experience in an *intra-group* structure are prematurely involved in *inter-group* activity. Often what they need is a positive *aggregate* experience rather than a premature attempt in a true group experience.

i.e.: team games, tournaments

Social skills necessary for this type of interaction are crucial for recreation programming. Those who do not have appropriate social skills within each of these groups will be unsuccessful in many recreation programs.

Selecting appropriate activities is dependent upon the abilities of the client participating in them. An important part of these skills is social in nature. The ability to interact successfully at each of the levels described by Avedon will be critical to the types of programs selected for the client.

The combination of the physical, cognitive, affective and social skills and abilities will therefore directly affect the selection of activities for a well balanced delivery of therapeutic recreation services.

An understanding of these skills and abilities will also enable the program planner to properly conduct activity analysis for those activities he selects. A work sheet designed for activity analysis can be found in Appendix III. Included on the form will be all necessary areas of analysis for activities. It is recommended that the program planner use this form with the activities he chooses for his program.

ACTIVITY ADAPTATION

Understanding or analyzing a particular activity will enable the program planner to adapt or modify the activity to meet the specific needs of his client population.

All or any of the impairments discussed above (physical, cognitive, affective or social) may affect the ability of the client to participate in certain activities. As a result, the program planner must be able to modify or adapt certain elements of an activity to ensure participation by his client. For example, a patient who wishes to join in a basketball game may be wheelchair bound. The basket may need to be lowered or a special basketball hoop for the floor may need to be used.

Many elements may be changed or adapted to meet the needs of the client. These include:

> The rules: i.e. changing the point system of a bowling game to make it easier to win.

> How to play the game: i.e. lowered basketball hoop or hoop on the floor.

> The goal of the activity: i.e. altering a craft project to facilitate easy results or achievement. In a painting class, an outline of the picture may be drawn to allow residents to paint within the lines. Thus, the goal is not the result of painting but the experience or joy of doing the painting.

Certain cautions must be taken to achieve successful activity adaptation. Viewing activity adaptation as a piece of clay may help the program planner mold it correctly.

First, too much change may lead to a new activity which may result in dissatisfaction for the client. Don't change the shape of the clay, simply mold it as needed! Don't change a basketball game into a bean bag toss because a patient cannot reach the basket. Lowering the basket or placing it closer to the patient will alter the activity but still allows for participation in a basketball game.

Second, adapt the activity or mold the clay *only where it needs to be molded*. Consideration of the client's specific impairment or limitation is crucial. The resident with impaired vision may require adaptation of a craft project to include brighter colored crayons or a clear outline of the drawing. If a part of the sculpture does not need adapting, simply leave it alone!

ACTIVITY CLASSIFICATION

Activity analysis and modification allow us to plan for and select appropriate activities for our specialized populations. These various activities may be classified into certain groups or general types. The Activities Supervisors Guide classifies these groups as follows.[5]

Social Activities

Social activities provide the opportunity for enjoyment and a pleasurable experience, usually within a loosely structured pattern. Social activities help decrease self consciousness by providing the opportunity for increased self-confidence. However, the program planner should be aware of the level of social interaction required for participation in socially oriented activities. This awareness will ensure successful participation by the client in appropriate social activities.

Diversional Activities

Some clients prefer activities which provide more than just an enjoyable experience. Diversional activities emphasize individual accomplishment which may be achieved by the client. Activities such as crafts projects may provide a feeling of accomplishment or self-fulfillment. However, activity adaptation may be necessary to achieve satisfying results for certain residents participating in diversional activities.

Work-Type Activities

Admission to long-term care facilities, especially for the elderly in nursing homes, often results in the loss of ones work role. Concomitant with this loss is a decreased feeling of importance and self-confidence. People therefore need a balance between work and play. Work type activities are a necessary component of therapeutic recreation services.

Volunteer Service Activities

Many clients need the opportunity of working but express the desire to "help others" in their work. Volunteer service activities are important ways of providing the "care receiver" with the opportunity to become the "care giver." Such activities may include clerical assistance, sorting and delivering mail or acting as a librarian or friendly visitor.

Intellectual Activities

As pointed out earlier, each part of one's personality affects the other. An active mind will provide the client with stimulation necessary for the functioning of the total person. Intellectual activities will also provide opportunities for ties to the outside world and community. Such activities include adult education courses, current events groups and discussion groups.

Religious and Spiritual Groups

All clients require the opportunity for religious self-expression provided by religious and spiritual activities. This becomes even more important with the elderly whose religious convictions tend to increase in later years.

Table 5-3: Activity Assessment Chart

Activity Name:	Activity Classification:	Social Interaction Level: (as identified by Avedon)	Behavioral Skills Required (numbered in order of importance)		
			Sensory Motor:	Cognitive:	Affective:
Adult Education	Intellectual	Unilateral	3	1	2
Bingo	Social	Aggregate	3	1	2
Board Games	Social	Inter-Ind.	3	1	2
Bowling	Social	Aggregate	1	2	3
Basketball	Social	Aggregate Intra-group Inter-group	1	3	2
Ceramics	Diversional	Aggregate	1	2	3
Current Events	Intellectual	Unilateral	3	1	2
Choral Group	Social	Intra-group	1	1	1
			(no one area is dominant)		
Card Games	Social	Multilateral	3	1	2
Dance Hour	Social	Intra-group	1	3	2
Drama	Intellectual	Intra-group	3	1	2
Exercise	Social	Aggregate	1	2	3
Knitting	Social	Aggregate	1	2	3
Movies	Intellectual	Aggregate	1	2	3
Music Appreciation	Intellectual	Aggregate	2	3	1
Painting	Diversional	Aggregate	1	3	2
Reading	Intellectual	Extra-ind.	2	1	3
Rhythm Band	Social	Intra-group	1	1	1
Sing-along	Social	Aggregate	1	2	3
Sheltered Work Shop	Work-type	Aggregate	2	1	3

The above Activity Assessment chart offers suggestions for specific recreation activities which may be used by the program planner. These activities may need to be analyzed or adapted for particular populations and are meant to serve as a possible resource for the activity director. By delineating the activity classification, its required interaction level and the behavioral skills needed for each activity, the program planner may be able to clarify which activities are appropriate for prospective clients.

The author provides additional suggested activities in Appendix VIII. The goals, objectives and procedures of each activity are outlined.

SUMMARY

Selecting activities is an important step in the program planning process. What seems to be an impressive list of recreation activities will have little meaning if the activities are inappropriate to the client being served. Activity analysis and modification are essential in providing worthwhile and meaningful activities for the client population being served.

Recognizing the skills and abilities necessary for activity participation through the behavioral arenas is important. Consideration of limitations in the sensory motor, cognitive and affective arenas will aid in program selection. The level of social interaction required by the activity and the client's social abilities must also be examined. The interactive processes which influence our behavior throughout each level of interaction need to be identified and considered.

Finally, activities require classification and adaptation to meet the needs of the diversified levels of physical and or psychological limitations of the institutionalized elderly population.

The total success of the activities program is dependent upon evaluation of that program. Evaluation will provide the program planner with information and assessments needed for improvement of the program. Chapter Six will address evaluation of program planning and implementation.

Chapter 6

PROGRAM EVALUATION

Evaluation Problems

One area which often seems neglected in therapeutic recreation is evaluation. Several factors seem to be responsible for the lack of evaluation in recreation programs.

First, many recreation directors are unfamiliar with the process of evaluation and their techniques. The complexity of certain evaluative methods or techniques also seems to frighten recreation professionals.

Second, the nature of recreation makes it difficult to obtain exact measurements. The number of clients attending a program does not necessarily reflect the success of the program. Satisfaction of the client, the feeling of joy one may experience with an activity, the individual growth of a client or the interpersonal relationships of the client during an activity are all much too difficult to evaluate in specific measurable terms. Further, the amount of joy or happiness experienced by one participant of an activity may be different for another participant of the same activity.

Third, a basic element of effective recreation programming is that of individual choice. Satisfaction of a recreation experience is achieved through participation on a voluntary basis, thereby limiting the use of certain evaluative methods or techniques. Thus, evaluation is often left to the observation and judgement of the activity leader rather than to results of specific tests.

Finally, many see evaluation as a time consuming, complicated task adding to the already existing problem of the paper work dilemma. The continued struggle of balancing required paper work with the direct service of activity programs is an obstacle faced by every activity director. The ignorance of the evaluation process and the burden it seems to present, at least partially account for its lack in recreation programming.

The need for increased use of evaluation is dependent upon an understanding of its influence on the total recreation program. Understanding the significance of evaluation in all areas may facilitate its use to a greater extent.

THE IMPORTANCE OF EVALUATION

The importance of the therapeutic recreation profession and its effects upon the total care of our client is finally being recognized. This recognition has brought with it a responsibility and accountability to our client and to all those professionals with whom we share the provision of such essential services.

An important part of this responsibility is the continued improvement of recreation programming which is the direct result of evaluation. The nature of long-term care facilities, especially nursing homes, is concomitant with changes which take place both in the community and in society at large. The changing population and admission of sicker, more frail elderly to our nursing homes, plays a crucial role in evaluating their needs for appropriate recreation services. Thus, evaluation in recreation makes it necessary to understand the social and cultural changes of our client brought about by society. Evaluating such changes on a continued basis will facilitate new and improved methods of recreation programming for our clients. A knowledge of where improvements or changes are needed will also enable easier planning for future goals and program achievements. Evaluation will therefore result in a more meaningful, effective level of recreation programming. This will also help to satisfy our accountability to quality assurance issues and outside regulatory agencies such as the state or other accreditation facilities. A high quality program through evaluation will also help rationalize our justification of services to administration whose necessary scrutiny over budgets is becoming more prevalent than ever before.

However, the effects of evaluation go beyond its primary function of program improvement. Every human being requires some type of recognition and or feedback while performing his job duties. Any program lacking feedback, evaluation or recognition of some type by the director will result in failure and poor staff morale.

Evaluation heightens awareness of one's objectives, providing direction and enabling the activity leader to determine how well he is acheiving the goals of his program. In addition, it becomes a learning process for the staff who in turn feel better about themselves and their jobs. Thus, accomplishment and the ability to grow as a professional will lead to increased morale within the activities department.

At The Jewish Home and Hospital for Aged, Bronx, New York, group program evaluation has proved to be highly successful both as an evaluative tool and for self-improvement of staff. Evaluation is utilized as a learning process, fostering group awareness and understanding of each other's goals and abilities. Evaluation is not seen as a vehicle for criticism but rather as an avenue of improvement for programming and staff leadership. Evaluation is carried out through the mutual understanding of one's talent and skill and the utilization of the therapeutic recreation process. This process has lead to a greater respect for each other's personal and professional growth and has resulted in a high regard for group cooperation and departmental morale. The actual method used for group program evaluations will be discussed later in the chapter. The forms used for this evaluation can be found in Appendix IV.

A knowledge of the role evaluation plays in therapeutic recreation should parallel a clear concept or understanding of what we mean by evaluation.

DEFINING EVALUATION

Of major significance to therapeutic recreation is the establishment of goals for our client, staff and programs. Equally important is the extent to which we achieve these goals. Evaluation is the process which determines how and if we are in fact achieving our stated goals.

Throughout the literature, evaluation is defined in a variety of ways. Patricia Farell sees evaluation as:

> a process whereby, through systematically judging, assessing and appraising the workings of a program, one gains information that indicates to programmers whether or not they are getting results or getting where they want to go . . . in sum, whether or not the program has value.[1]

Gunn and Peterson refer to evaluation as a "method of documenting operations and outcomes to determine the strengths and weaknesses of the program."[2]

Evaluation is therefore a process which enables the program planner to assess or determine the value of various aspects of the activities program, thereby facilitating necessary improvements in all areas.

TYPES OF EVALUATION

Evaluation can be as simple as one wishes or as complex as necessary. Scientific techniques may be used to appraise or measure a specific program while evaluation may also be done to appraise the achievement of the overall goals or general objectives.

Evaluation may be done intermittently, evaluating for achievement of objectives, or may be utilized by systematically evaluating each component before moving on to the next activity or stage.

Another type of evaluation which the activity leader should be familiar with is formative evaluation. This is an on-going evaluation used to determine the program's accomplishments so that improvements can be made. Through the compiling of data, information is provided which allows the program planner to make changes during the entire program planning process.

Finally, summative evaluation appraises or evaluates the accomplishments of the program. The use of certain procedures obtained through studies helps draw conclusions regarding the program's effectiveness or accomplishments.

Regardless of the type of evaluation being used, it should be understood that evaluation is part of the total process of program planning. Evaluation needs to be built into the entire recreation process to ensure that each step is appropriately appraised for achievement of goals. Evaluation is therefore the result of a carefully planned process which begins with analysis and moves along the continuum of program planning, goal setting, implementation and evaluation.

Gunn and Peterson concur that program evaluation is part of program planning. In relation to the leisure ability approach, they outline four sequential steps:[3]

1. Conceptualize the specific program.
2. Design the program including terminal program objectives, enabling objectives, performance measures, and the content and process for each enabling objective.
3. Develop the implementation plan.
4. Design the evaluation.

Thus, evaluation should be included as an essential step in the total process of program planning. Evaluation is not a footnote to program planning.

Effective evaluation requires that all necessary information (data, procedures, etc.) be determined at the very beginning of the program planning process. Ignoring evaluation through the entire process of program planning will eliminate important information, making it difficult to evaluate at an effective level.

The actual process of evaluation may be carried out in a variety of ways. The literature indicates the availability of several models for evaluation.

EVALUATION MODELS

David Austin, in his book, Therapeutic Recreation Processes and Techniques, presents two models which are commonly used in therapeutic recreation. First, he describes the Tylerian Model which defines evaluation as:

> a process utilizing the scientific approach for determining the congruence between stated objectives and actual behavior during summative evaluation.[4]

Based upon this definition, the model examines actual outcomes to see if they match sought outcomes. Thus, discrepancies pinpoint areas for investigation. The identification of these discrepancy areas will allow for change and program development.

Gunn and Peterson also identify this type of evaluation as "discrepancy evaluation." In relation to the systems designed approach, discrepancy evaluation is concerned with three areas: inputs, process and outcomes.[5] Again, the intended outcomes will be compared to the actual outcomes in each of these three areas.

Input

Gunn and Peterson identify the following five areas as the input of a therapeutic recreation program: "staff, clients, supplies, facilities and funding."[6] Each of these areas will need to be evaluated: examining and comparing the planned input with the actual input. Discrepancies in any of these areas will result in program change and improvements. The following are some questions the author suggests which may help the evaluator examine each input area, determining if the intended outcomes equal the actual outcomes.

Staff

1. Are specific staff skills required (crafts, music etc.) to help client accomplish necessary program objectives?
2. Is there specific training required to help client accomplish program objectives? Does the staff require training for specific treatment modalities such as reality orientation, sensory stimulation, behavior modification?
3. Is the personality or nature of staff appropriate to the needs of the elderly population?
4. Does the staff personality facilitate communication between client and worker?

Client

Is the client population appropriate for the goals of the program as designed?

1. Have the physical limitations of the client been considered in planning the program?
2. Have the emotional factors been appropriately considered in planning the program?
3. Have the mental and intellectual abilities of the client been considered appropriately?
    i.e. Has an adult education class been planned with clients who are confused or disoriented?
4. Has the program been planned without regard to the interest of the client?
    i.e. Has an opera group been implemented for those who do not enjoy music?

Supplies

Supplies are an important part of the program planning process. Evaluation of supplies is required as a possible discrepancy area.

1. Are the appropriate supplies available for the activity planned?
    i.e. Are musical instruments available for a rhythm band?
2. Are the supplies adequate for the number of participants?
    i.e. Has a game hour been planned with a limited supply of games?
3. Are the supplies being used appropriately to the physical needs of the client?
    i.e. Is a 10-pound bowling ball being used for a frail elderly person?
4. Are supplies appropriate to the mental and or intellectual needs of the client?
    i.e. Are games too difficult for the client to understand?

Facilities

Available facilities must be evaluated for possible discrepancies between actual and intended outcomes.

1. Are the available facilities adequate for the type of activity being implemented?

> i.e.   Is the auditorium large enough for a birthday party or entertainment?

Is there an adequate number of chairs and tables in the crafts room?

2.   Are the facilities available appropriate for use with the client and activity program?
> i.e.   Are the chairs or couches in the lounge areas appropriate for elderly population to use?

Funding

Funding must also be evaluated for possible discrepancies.

1.   Is there adequate funding for the type of activities planned?
> i.e.   Is there enough money to hire a teacher for an adult education class?

2.   Is there money for supplies for activities?
> i.e.   Has bingo been planned without money to purchase prizes or bingo cards?

All of the input areas must be evaluated to be sure that the program has been implemented as designed.

Process

In the systems designed approach outlined by Gunn and Peterson, Process represents the activities described during the program plan. Here, two areas of concern are identified.[7]

1.   Were the designated content and process followed?
2.   Were the activities and processes that were implemented appropriate and useful in achieving the objectives?

Thus, the areas of discrepancy will be identified to facilitate change and improvements.

Outcomes

Within the systems designed approach, the evaluator also examines whether achievement of objectives have been reached by the client. The discrepancy model will therefore identify which areas need revisions or change. To effect change or improvements it will also be necessary to examine what areas of the program may have prevented the accomplishment of its goals or objectives.

Although the discrepancy model offers an approach which seems logical and systematic, Austin points out some possible problems inherent in its application.[8]

First, there may be a tendency to establish only those program objectives which are easily measured. Thus, other important outcomes may be ignored by failing to establish those program objectives which are more difficult to measure. Program objectives related to the affective arena may be ignored because they are more difficult to measure than those of the cognitive arena.

Another problem may be that of establishing "valid and comprehensive" program objectives. Certain critical objectives must be included or information concerning the progress toward the stated objectives will be of little value. As Austin notes, if a sports club does not include an objective which deals with sportsmanship, any evaluation will be of questionnable value, regardless of the other objectives being appraised.[9]

Third, the discrepancy model does not concern itself with unplanned outcomes which often occur in recreation programs. As Austin indicates, some of the most important outcomes are those that are unplanned but seem to evolve as a natural outcome of the recreation experience. For example, an unplanned outcome of a drama group may be the strong sense of belonging or respect developed between each participant. Although this was not planned for, a new program objective may now be established.

Finally, this type of evaluation does not consider information or data such as attendance patterns or participation among its participants.

Another model discussed by Austin is the "Naturalistic Model."[10] This model, whose scope is broader than the discrepancy model, examines program activities and objectives. It goes beyond merely stating program objectives as it examines what happens during the program. Further, it recognizes the elements which may have influenced the program.

Inherent in this evaluation model is the examination of interpersonal, social and cultural variables that surround behavior. Thus, the context of the situation is also considered. This model is therefore less scientific than other evaluation models.

Examining the variety of evaluation models indicates that program evaluation goes beyond its concern for "quantitative data" and the program objectives. Program evaluation should ecnompass more than the measurement of objectives.

QUALIFICATIONS OF EVALUATORS

Effective evaluation necessitates certain qualifications or competencies which the evaluator should possess. These should include an understanding of:

the underlying principles and procedures which formulate concepts of therapeutic recreation.

the areas which require evaluation such as leadership, programming and facilities.

the characteristics of evaluation and the use of scientific and non-scientific evaluative methods.

utilization and implementation of appropriate instruments used to measure evaluative situations.

i.e.   Often, evaluators incorrectly use certain factors in measuring the success of programs. Attendance records have often been used to prove the success of an activity or to show its support for the program. When using attendance records as the sole instrument of measurement, the results will be unrealistic. Additional data will be required for the evaluative process.

information and data which help determine selection of appropriate evaluative techniques.

the results of evaluation and the ability to interpret data, measurements and the level of success or failures related to the predetermined goals and objectives.

EVALUATION APPROACHES

A variety of evaluation models permeate the literature. Regardless of the model used, an understanding of the approaches used for evaluation is an important consideration. Evaluation does not necessarily have to represent scientific techniques. A combination of simple appraisals as well as scientific methods will provide adequate evaluation.

Control Groups

One scientific approach is the use of control groups. As previously discussed, the nature of recreation often makes it difficult to obtain exact measurements of successful participation in activities. However, observation of patient behavior often provides information and data useful to program evaluation. In addition to achievement of goals or performance level, it is important to recognize the degree to which certain behaviors may have changed, thereby indicating some success with the recreation program. The degree to which positive behavioral changes are accomplished will help determine how effective a program may be.

To measure this, a control group may be established which is unrelated to the program. Each group would be measured to see if the group involved in the program has achieved more significant behavioral changes than the group not involved in the program. We can also measure how much change took place in the participating group by measuring their characteristics before and after the program.

For example, a pilot program was established on three skilled nursing units of The Jewish Home and Hospital for Aged, Bronx, New York. A specific staff member conducted activity programming on these units at the same specified hours five days a week. Specialized programming designed for the regressed SNF population was implemented. Although activity programs occurred in the remaining units of the facility, they were not exposed to the specialized activities implemented at the specified hours five days a week. Behavioral observations of residents of all units were observed and noted previous to implementation of the pilot program. Utilizing the remaining units as the control group, the results seemed to indicate the following for the pilot program units.

1. A greater degree of verbalization occurred with residents on the pilot program.

2. An increase in "appropriate communication" occurred, that is, statements on behaviors that related to the activity situation which took place.

3. A greater account of concentration within the activity seemed to occur.

4. The resident appeared to be calmer. In some instances, medications were decreased.

Standards as Evaluation

Evaluation by standards involves the establishment of specific criteria or measurements upon which the evaluation can be compared to the achieved level of performance. Standards are usually established to ensure the client a certain degree of performance and a high quality of programming. In addition, they provide an accountability against which a system of program effectiveness can be measured. Finally, achievement of standards often leads to accreditation by certain regulatory agencies.[11]

The New York State department of Mental Health is responsible for maintaining the standards set by the New York State Hospital code. These standards set in response to many of the reasons stated above, have great implications for the delivery of therapeutic recreation services in long-term care facilities. The standards established affect several areas of recreation including:

1. Philosophy and goals of the recreation program.
2. Number of staff required for delivery of services.
3. Types of programs delivered.

4. Frequency of program delivery (seven days a week programming is required in New York State)

5. Documentation of programming effectiveness upon resident population.

These standards are measured during state surveys through a series of lists, observations and interviews of both residents and staff. Although this type of evaluation tool can be easily utilized, certain problems are also presented.

Standards used as evaluations often imply that they are equal in importance. Although certain aspects of the activity program are more important than others, they tend to be viewed equally by some standards.[12] In addition, these standards often focus on concrete areas which are evaluated in numbers. Attendance records and frequency of activities often seem to be more important in satisfying established standards, a fact which ignores the positive effects of certain programs upon the population being served.

When using standards as an evaluation approach, all areas should be adequately covered. Clear and concise criteria should be available for each standard.

Howard Danford offers five steps which he considers basic to any effective approach to evaluation.[13]

1. Prepare a clear statement of the goals you seek through the recreation program.
    Goals are basic to any evaluation. Without them, there will be no way of evaluating your progress or what you have achieved.

2. Interpret these goals, whenever possible, in terms of the behavior of people.
    Identify the kinds of behavior that indicate progress toward achievement of this specific goal. In a nursing home, you may want to improve the social skill of sharing with others. Identifying this type of behavior within recreation activities would indicate the progress toward the desired goal.

3. Provide the kinds of recreation situation or experiences which lead to the established goals. In a nursing home activity program, increased sharing skills through participation in a cooking class will provide appropriate recreation experiences.

4. Observe the behavior of the participants in terms of the previously prepared list of behaviors which will indicate progress of goal achievement.

5. Analyze the results of your study; attempt to discover basic causes for our failures and successes and make the changes in your program which seem to be indicated.

Evaluation by Objectives

The amount of enjoyment or pleasure one derives from participating in recreation experience depends upon each individual participant. Further, it is extremely difficult to measure the enjoyment received. Thus, the recreation leader often relies on observations and subjective judgements.

Often, the recreation activity is also measured inaccurately by how much is spent on the activity or how many people attend. It becomes essential, then, to utilize every means possible in evaluating the recreation program.

Evaluation by objectives necessitates evaluation of all areas such as the program, staff, participants and the facilities. Sound evaluation will result in revision of objectives relating to these program areas.

In evaluation by objectives, Farell points to consideration of two types:[14]

1. The broad objectives for the program itself.
2. The specific behavioral objectives for the participants.

Thus, as Farell indicates, the broad goals formulated for the program itself must be transposed into specific participant objectives which can be measured. Measurement of the degree to which we achieve our objectives will therefore enable the program planner to institute necessary changes.

Evaluation Procedures

A variety of evaluative techniques have been used in recreation including simple appraisal methods and the use of scientific methods.

As John Hutchinson states, these techniques which are used to compile data on recreation factors comprise evaluative procedures. These procedures fall into two general categories: quantitative and qualitative.[15]

A quantitative procedure refers to the use of measurement tools utilized to collect specific numbers and data for evaluation purposes. The data collected represent information to be used with additional factors which require accurate evaluation. Evaluating the fact that only 10 people attend a movie as a recreation activity will have little significance if other factors such as the poor quality of the movie or the inappropriate title are not considered.

The use of quantitative data are not enough in recreation. Qualitative procedures may need to be used as well. The use of observations, description of programs, questionnaires, sociograms, interviews, surveys or lists comprise qualitative data. These techniques should be used when more scientific tools are not available.

Measurement Tools

Determining the appropriate procedures for evaluation depends upon the tools used. These tools contain certain qualities or traits. Without these qualities (reliability, validity and objectivity), evaluating the results may lead to inaccurate conclusions.

Validity. Validity implies that the procedure appraises what it sets out to appraise. A test which adds the number of participants attending a weekly cooking class would not be a valid measuring instrument of the number of residents who actually participated in cooking a recipe in the class.

Reliability. The procedure or tool used must be reliable or dependable. This means that the application of a test will yield equal results when carried out under the same conditions. Thus, will the ability of the elderly drama group participant to recite his lines be repeated consistently on different days or will each test yield different results? The evaluator must be aware of outside factors which may influence the reliability of the test. These may include the fact that the resident may not feel well or may not be interested in that activity on that day. The mood of his fellow residents or the death of a peer on a particular day may also influence the reliability of a test or procedure.

Objectivity. With an objective procedure, the evaluator does not impose his own bias or subjective judgement upon the measuring tool. Measuring an ingredient of a recipe in a cooking class by comparing it to the amount of a similar ingredient would be using subjective evidence. Thus, the use of a measuring bowl would offer more objective results.

Measurement Tools

Certain measuring instruments are especially appropriate for evaluation in recreation. Farell and Lundergren have identified the following as some of these instruments.[16] For a detailed discussion on the development of such measuring instruments, the author suggests referring to *Process of Recreation Programming: Theory and Techniques* by Farell and Lundergren.

Questionnaires. These are tools used to help the recreation leader acquire information needed for evaluation and assessment of the client. They may be used for a variety of reasons and are usually conducted through interview format.

The type of questions utilized may be multiple choice, fill in, true or false, checklists or open-ended questions.

The use of questionnaires for obtaining information regarding recreation preferences and interests is very common in nursing homes and long-term care facilities. Questionnaires provide pertinent background information and help collect data essential to the program planner.

Information regarding recreation interests, prior lifestyle, social outlets and voluntary activities help the planner evaluate the needs of his client in determining an individualized activities program and treatment plan. (See Chapter Ten, "The Paper Work Dilemma," for more details concerning the Activity Preference Questionnaire).

Observations.   These are specific procedures which record or evaluate certain outcomes or behaviors. Evaluators using observations need to demonstrate objectivity both in their behavior assessment and in their recordings.

Observations are probably one of the most commonly used evaluation procedures in recreation. Due to the nature of recreation activities, observations may be done with or without the patient being aware of this process. As discussed earlier, observations are utilized as a successful measurement tool for program evaluation at The Jewish Home and Hospital for Aged.

A specially designed program evaluation form (see Appendix IV) is used to observe program leadership, resident behavior and staff interaction. This tool is used by the activity director as well as with the entire activities staff during group program evaluation.

Programs conducted by each activity leader are observed and evaluated by the director on a regularly scheduled basis, once a month jointly by the entire activity staff. Using the group program evaluation tool, observations are recorded for each activity observed. These observations and evaluations are critiqued and discussed further at regularly scheduled staff meetings.

Involvement of all activity staff for group program evaluations facilitates groups cohesiveness and input. In addition, direct involvement of the activity staff fosters a greater interest among all concerned.

Sociograms.   These are graphic pictures which display group structure. They identify relationships among the group members and indicate social relationships such as pairs, cliques, etc. by asking questions. The response to a question such as, "Who would you like to sit next to at a barbecue?" may be presented graphically as a sociogram.

Great emphasis is placed upon the social acceptance or rejection of individuals participating in a recreation experience. Therapeutic recreation is often a means through which behavioral change will culminate in social acceptance of a group situation.

Sociometry is a scientific technique which studies the organization of groups, determining the nature of the structure within the group. A sociometric test identifies those who may be accepted or popular, those who may be rejected or those who may be disliked.

Howard Danford indicates the following values of sociometric techniques.[17]

1. Improving the social adjustment of the individual:

   Identifying patterns of acceptance or rejection through sociometric techniques allows the activity leader to help facilitate changes of behavior with those who need help in group structures. This technique also helps to point out or identify those with leadership abilities. Thus, appropriate skills can be developed by the activity leader to help foster leadership qualities.

2. Improving group relations:

   Sociometric techniques help identify areas of tension, hostility or friction within group situations. Identifying problem areas of interpersonal relations will provide the activity leader with the opportunity of correcting these socially ineffective situations.

3. Improving the organization of groups:

   Most groups work best when a cooperative effort is evident. Groups whose individuals are fighting or competing with each other will have little success. Sociometric techniques identify individuals with similar personalities and tastes, thereby fostering group cohesiveness.

Areas of Evaluation

Evaluation of the total program includes leadership, programming and facilities.

Leadership. The effect of leadership upon the success of recreation is of great importance. Although leadership and evaluation will be discussed in a separate chapter ("The Use of Effective Leadership"), it is necessary to offer a brief review of leadership evaluation at this point.

Leadership evaluation is the measurement of the degree to which we have successfully achieved established objectives. The results of these appraisals will lead to the revision of certain methods and objectives. Evaluation helps identify problem areas which necessitate change. As Shivers explains:

> The objective of examining the results of leadership is to determine whether goals have been accomplished; the objective of examining techniques is to determine whether certain methods are being followed. The reason for comparing outcome with technique is to determine whether the technique should be changed in some way.[18]

The success of any group depends upon the achievements of objectives facilitated by the leader. Thus, evaluating the leader is an essential task. Since most evaluation of leadership is subjective in nature, there is no standard set of measurements which can be applied. However, many variables effect the use of these tools. As Shivers laments, the "best indicator of leadership may be the pragmatic approach, i.e. does it lead to success?"[19] However, as he indicates, the problem with this approach is the definition of success. What may be success for one may not be defined as success for another. Therefore, leadership should be considered from the point of view of the leader, the participant, the agency and the evaluator.[20]

Participant. The participant of the group is dependent upon the leader for achieving his goals or needs. Thus, as Shivers notes, the level or degree to which the participant achieves his desires is a good indication of the success of the leader.

The elderly participant who receives satisfaction and an enjoyable experience through participating in a group activity, will probably indicate a high level of success for his leader. When the participant likes his leader and believes in the goals of the group, he is more willing to participate in such activities. The elderly participant is often heard stating: "I'm only in this group because of you (the leader)."

Agency. The agency will also evaluate the success of the leader. The agency will be concerned with how well the director through his leadership achieves the goals and needs of the agency. Successful leadership for the agency will depend upon what is produced. Most agencies provide mechanisms for evaluation of the recreation director. In some cases, evaluation is directly related to salary increases.

The leader. His success will be determined by the degree to which his participant achieves his goals or needs. If he is successful in his leadership, he will have gained the trust and acceptance of those in his group. Finally, the leader's success will be evident if the participant is willing to remain in the group.

The recreation director. The recreation director or administrator is responsible for the planning and implementation of the total recreation program. He must be able to coordinate the planning, organizing, follow up, delegation of responsibilities and communicating with others inside and out of the department.

The success of the director will be determined by the degree to which he accomplishes his tasks or objectives in all of these areas. Evaluation will help determine where improvements or changes are indicated. The activity director should be evaluated at least annually by the administrator or executive director of his agency.

Facilities and areas. The most well planned activity program will be almost impossible to implement without appropriate facilities and areas with which to conduct activities. These areas need to be evaluated for their size, use, accessibility and safety.

First, an adequate number of activity rooms (auditorium, large and small group rooms) must be available to service the client population involved in the program.

Second, the room available should be accessible to those attending activities. A large sized, beautifully decorated auditorium would be useless if the residents of a nursing home could not reach the auditorium easily or without great assistance.

Third, the furniture and equipment in the rooms need to be evaluated for their appropriateness. Large chairs or couches which make it difficult for the elderly to sit in or get out of would certainly be inappropriate.

Fourth, the safety of the rooms needs to be considered. Rooms should not be cluttered. Easy access to and from the room especially for wheelchairs and walkers should be available.

Finally, can the room be used for more than one purpose and should it be evaluated for this possibility?

Summary

The importance of evaluation and its effects upon program improvement, staff feedback and recognition cannot be overemphasized.

Without evaluation, there will be no tools available for measurement of the successes or failures of the total recreation program. Hence, it is imperative that evaluation be viewed as part of the "total" process of program planning and be built into the planning and implementation stages.

A clear understanding of what is meant by evaluation as well as its types and approaches are necessary. Evaluation procedures should include the use of measurement tools and the scientific and non-scientific techniques necessary for program evaluation.

Finally, the program planner must maintain an awareness of the appropriate areas for evaluation. Without continued evaluation of the leadership, the participant, the facilities and the programs, the delivery of therapeutic recreation services will suffer the consequences of a stagnated and benign program.

Chapter 7

THE USE OF EFFECTIVE LEADERSHIP

Understanding therapeutic recreation, developing a goal and philosophy and creating a well balanced program are all essential ingredients of a successful activities program.

However, the use of effective leadership is required to help guide the integration of these ingredients into a successful program. Without an effective leader these ingredients will be of little value. As Danford states:

> Leadership is by far the most important single factor in the successful operation of a program of recreation. Without good leadership no recreation department can succeed regardless of the many other assets it may possess.[1]

THE MEANING OF LEADERSHIP

The realm of leadership consists of more than the "recreation leader" who directs activities in the recreation program. Definitions of leadership abound throughout the literature. J. Tillman Hall sees leadership as:

> the ability to stimulate, guide and direct others; if it is constructive leadership the direction is desirable and approved by the group. A leader has influence because others follow him and his advice.[2]

Keith Davis describes leadership as:

> the ability to persuade others to seek defined objectives enthusiastically.

It is the human factor which binds a group together and motivates it toward goals.[3]

Leadership is therefore a process by which the leader helps move its group toward the achievement of stated goals. Several variables influence leadership and the success of goal achievement.

Danford believes three factors or conditions must be present before leadership can exist:[4]

1. a group of two or more persons.

2. goals or common tasks to be pursued.

3. at least some of the group members must have different responsibilities; where all have the same duties no leader exists.

LEADERSHIP THEORIES

Inherent in all of these definitions is the fact that leadership involves human behavior and social interactions with others. Many studies have been done regarding the variables which affect and influence the emergence of leadership. Previous to examining "recreation leadership," it is important to understand the basic concepts which underlie the theories of leadership.

The Trait Theory

Previous to the belief that leadership was a result of one's behavior and his relation to a group situation, the Trait Theory was based upon the belief that leaders were born with specific traits. It was these traits which were thought to be a common thread among all leaders which provided man with the opportunity of rising to a leadership position. A prominent belief was that those who maintain leadership traits or characteristics would naturally evolve into leaders. However, several studies began to show that specific traits or identifiable qualities were not common to *all* leaders. Ralph Stodgdill further disproved any consistant traits characterizing *all* leaders:

> A person does not become a leader by virtue of the possession of some combination of traits, but the pattern of personal characteristics of the leader must bear some relevant relationship to the characteristics, activities and goals of the followers. Their leadership must be conceived in terms of an interaction of variables which are in constant flux and change.[5]

In spite of the above, the research did show that certain traits appeared more often than others. As a result, certain generalizations were made which seemed to indicate that qualities related to sociability, motivation and ability were evident more often among groups of leaders than among members of the group. H. Bonner also suggests that specific traits do seem to appear in certain leaders. However, he also notes that group-dynamic investigations suggest that it is not the trait which specifically contributes to the leader, but the relationship of all the factors which influence the group structure at a certain time.[6] Thus, determining leadership cannot be based solely upon certain traits or qualities.

The Group Function Theory

The continued research which disproved the Trait Theory resulted in a new approach to leadership. This theory suggests a shift of leadership properties from the person to the group. With this shift comes the responsibility of every member of the group to contribute in some way to its goals or achievements. The contribution of each individual is seen as a leadership role. The use of individual leadership traits is therefore determined by the purpose or function of the group. Changes within the group may warrant leaders with different traits. In addition, as conditions change, leadership responsibility may shift to different members of the group. Thus, the leadership role of each member becomes the catalyst in bringing about goal achievement.

Leadership as a group function has sparked some debate among researchers. Some believe that goal achievement requires the concentrated effort of a select group of leaders, while others feel that any action taken toward goal achievement by any members may be considered leadership roles. Whatever the case may be, it is important to note that this approach does not eliminate the function of a qualified leader. The individual leader is therefore an important part of the group. Thus, according to the Group Function Theory of leadership, individuals play a key role in shaping the group and determining leadership composition. The ability of the leader to influence its group members further supports the significance of the role of each individual leader. Thus, the individual leader has an important role and definite effect upon the group.

The Group Function Theory offers significant considerations for the program planner. It is important for the recreation leader to inspire leadership and promote independence among his client whenever possible. For example, resident councils facilitate group leadership, encouraging residents to accept leadership tasks.

Dependent upon the needs of the resident council as a group, each resident may accept leadership responsibilities (i.e. floor captains, committee chairpersons), thereby contributing to the group's overall goal or objectives.

Another opportunity for group leadership exists in certain recreation activities which should be examined by the program planner. Residents may be given responsibility for leading exercise groups, sing-alongs, etc., thereby sharing responsibilities among all members of the group.

The Situational Theory

Further research studies began to indicate that the situation in which individuals were found had a direct influence upon their emergence as leaders. This theory suggests that the leader must be able to solve problems specifically related to the group. Specific qualities or traits were required to help the group solve its problem or achieve its goals. Leadership qualities which did not relate to the group situation were ineffective in solving the group's problems. Thus, as the situation changes, new leaders may emerge within the same group.

This theory has great implications for recreation. First, it is extremely important for the recreation leader conducting group programs to have qualities or traits which relate to the needs of his group. A recreation leader may be trained as a dance therapist or may be an enthusiastic leader of an exercise class. However, his personal qualities or abilities may not be as successful in leading a cooking group or arts and crafts class. Just as one leader may have qualities which influence or facilitate worthy discussion groups, this same leader may fail at leading a singalong. It therefore becomes crucial for the program planner to be able to assign the appropriate leader to his group. Thus, specific qualifications or traits of the recreation leader will be demanded by the situation of the group to be conducted.

We must therefore afford every opportunity for staff education and growth which will help facilitate leadership traits or qualities. Finally, the leader must be able to communicate with the group about its situation and goals. He must instill a sense of security and must be accepted by his group members.

LEADERSHIP STYLES

Fred Fiedler has made a significant contribution to leadership behavior. Through his development of the LPC scale (least preferred co-worker) he was able to measure leadership styles and movement toward the satisfaction of group goals.[7] The LPC scale allowed Fiedler to identify two distinct leadership styles: the high LPC person who "derived his major satisfactions from successful interpersonal relationship, and the low LPC person who derives his major satisfactions from task performances."[8] According to Fiedler, the difference in effectiveness of these two leadership styles was dependent upon the situation. However, he indicated the requirements of three variables before leadership effectiveness could be measured:[9]

1. The leader's personal relations with group members—how much the leader is liked and admired.
2. The organizational structure of the group—the way duties and responsibilities for each member of the group are assigned.
3. The leader's actual power or authority.

Therefore, as Shivers notes, under the correct conditions, either type of leadership may be effective. However, it is important to recognize that whatever style is utilized, certain goals need to be achieved by the group. It is often difficult to achieve these goals when criticism is warranted yet group support is required. Thus, as experience shows, effective leadership usually requires a degree of depersonalization of relationships in order to achieve task objectives.

Perhaps one of the most significant contributions to leadership styles was made by Ralph White and Ronald Lippe under the supervision of Kurt Lewin. They studied groups of young boys involved in after school activities. Each of the groups was composed of five children exposed to different leadership styles which included the autocratic and the democratic styles. The children were composed of groups with similar IQ's, popularity, etc. Through the study, a third style emerged as another form of democratic style called "laissez-faire." The objectives of the study included:[10]

1. To study the effects on group and individual behavior of three experimental variations in adult leadership.
2. To study the group and individual relations to shifts from one type of leadership to another within the same group.
3. To seek relationship between the nature and content of other group memberships.

Autocratic Leadership

In this group the leader became the dominant figure, making all assignments and decisions on his own without any input from his group members. His autocratic leadership involved little interaction with the group members.

The results from this group indicated that the children had difficulty in completing tasks independently. They exhibited greater dependence and less creativity. In the absence of the leader, some children became disruptive.

Democratic Leadership

In this group, leadership fostered cooperation and group cohesiveness. The leader made decisions based upon the input of those in the group. The goals of the group were clarified and expectations were clearly specified. Group members selected their own partners and leaders worked closely with all of them offering directions along the way.

The results from this group indicated more creativity and a more genuine or sincere interest in the group. Greater independence and less aggressive behavior was observed.

Laissez-Faire Leadership

In this group, little leadership was offered. Members were allowed to do as they pleased. The results indicated dissatisfaction with this group. Little work was accomplished and little satisfaction was achieved.

These studies seem to indicate the need for democratic leadership in the recreation situation. The success of any group is dependent upon the accomplishments of goals or objectives, and the growth and satisfacion of its members.

A word of caution is required here. It is important to consider not only the leadership types but the situation of the group. The recreation activities of a long-term care facility seem to be most appropriatetly conducted by the democratic leader. However, special considerations of the elderly often require certain decisions which may need to be made by the leader. Physical and or psychological limitations may therefore affect the group situation.

Just as group theories seem to have evolved over time, so will new research probably exhibit further changes. Although each theory and leadership style seems to offer its own contribution, no one single theory or style seems to be responsible for the theory of leadership behavior.

The foundation of all leadership is the ability to establish trust and acceptance by its group members. Just as the recreation leader aims to achieve acceptance of his group, the administrator must also create an atmosphere of trust and acceptance among his department heads, directors and staff.

Good leadership provides the opportunity for members to make suggestions and this in turn plays a significant role in the achievement of the agency's goals. Direct involvement by staff members creates greater interest and more effort toward goal achievement. The principles of the democratic process facilitate communication necessary for the exchange of ideas among staff members and residents alike.

Whether the ideas offered are accepted or not, it is crucial for the staff or the residents to be involved in the decision making process. This communication and exchange of ideas also adds to group cohesiveness as the group members identify more easily with the ideas they have made. Thus, through the democratic process, direct involvement of group members will lead to greater cooperation and higher group morale.

In addition, the success of any group rests upon the ability of its members to work together. We must remind ourselves that *every* staff member of the long-term care facility shares a common goal: to provide a holistic approach to the care of our clients. The needs of our clients demand our attention every minute of our busy day. We often get caught in the trap of trying to solve our problems without involving other departments. We tend to lose sight of the fact that we should be working together, combining our resources in an effort toward achieving our common goal. We sometimes need to forego our personal goals for group goals.

Leadership is, therefore, found at every level of the hierarchy in the long-term care facility. The interpersonal process is essential toward establishing relationships which will enable the functioning of the group to achieve both its departmental and agency's goals.

UNDERSTANDING HUMAN BEHAVIOR: INTERPERSONAL RELATIONSHIPS

The functioning of groups depends upon the interpersonal relationships of its members. Leadership requires an understanding of these interpersonal relationships or the personality factors and behaviors which precipitate responses of people.

Self-image or self-concept is probably one of the key factors which affects our behavior. Self-image is built upon years of experiences and interactions which influence the development of our identity and values. The development of one's self-image becomes the essential factor in determining our behavior patterns. Dennis Waitly believes:

> Our self-image determines the kind of person we are. We see ourselves and create our own self-image based upon every thought, triumph or loss we experience. Every event in our environment and our lives contributes to the development of our self-image.[11]

In addition, the self-image helps determine how others react toward us. As Norman Cameron suggests:

> The self-image represents one's status as an organism, as a unit in a series with social systems (family group, neighborhood group, school, religious and work groups) as a person toward whom, within the different social systems mentioned, other people have many different and conflicting attitudes, and toward whom the person himself has his own complex attitudes.[12]

Thus, throughout our lives, we respond to the stimuli of our surrounding environment. Some of these stimuli may be negative, representing reactions or responses of others toward us. These pressures necessitate the maintenance and protection of our own self-image and self-concept, thereby directly influencing our behavioral responses. In light of these continued internal and external pressures, defense mechanisms are employed to facilitate our functioning level at the highest possible degree. It is important to briefly describe some of these mechanisms, since they represent behavioral forms which affect how group members will behave and interact. Thus, an awareness of these mechanisms will help the leader understand why certain behaviors occur, thereby facilitating appropriate leadership techniques.

Frustration

Frustration occurs when the client is faced with a problem and cannot achieve his goal. The person's response will sometimes elicit anger while at other times withdrawal may occur. Thus, the elderly participant of a recreation group who is having difficulty completing a project or who has a physical or psychological problem may become angry or even withdraw from the activity.

Sublimation

Sublimation is the transformation of certain actions or energies into socially acceptable modes of behavior. For example, the elderly resident who is angry at her roommate, may take a part in the drama club to act our her frustrations on the stage.

Denial

Denial usually occurs when a person denies something he perceives. A typical denial response may be: "Oh, that can't be true." Denial may also occur when someone ignores a particular situation. This type of defense mechanism has been seen in unhappy adults.

The recreation leader working in the long-term care facility has an advantage in that he will probably work with the same groups of people for a longer period of time than those in other health care settings. An understanding of the kinds of behavior which begin to appear through the group process will be essential toward achieving effective leadership. Recognition of these defense mechanisms and behavioral patterns are not always easily identified. However a knowledge of human behavior is essential for communication and effective leadership. More importantly, the therapeutic recreation specialist must be able to identify certain behaviors if we wish to be able to change them through the therapeutic recreation process.

Understanding Group Dynamics

Group dynamics is the understanding of the group structure, its nature and role and how it funtions. Through group dynamics we hope to understand how groups affect its members and how members affect the group situation. Through an understanding of human behavior and group dynamics we begin to see how certain relationships develop which affect both the individual and the group situation.

The group (a set of interrelated individuals) becomes a process through which its members interact to achieve a goal. Through this interaction behaviors will change. Thus, every member becomes interrelated and is dependent upon the entire group for its satisfaction and goal achievement. Of equal importance is the identification and sense of belonging we exhibit to the group.

As stated earlier, group dynamics refers to group functions. It is important for the effective leader to understand the variables or characteristics of the group.

Group Cohesiveness

An important function of the group is the achievement of goals which are often difficult to obtain outside of the group. Group cohesiveness has been seen as the elements which help keep the members "together," functioning as a group. Common ideals of a group whose members have similar goals will probably lead to a strong group cohesiveness. A group of residents who share a common interest in music and are members of a choral group will probably have a strong group cohesivenss. Thus, the behavior of the individual which coincides with the norms or values of the group adds to the cohesiveness of the group.

Group Norms

The norms are the values or customs which guide or determine the expected behavior of the group. These values are ideas usually acquired through years of experiences related to contacts with families, peers, and other group associations. When the behavior of the group deviates from its norms, there will be a breakdown of cohesiveness. Thus, when group norms are not adhered to, certain sanctions or punishments may exist to prevent the group from disolving. When group norms are adhered to, individual and group goals are more easily achieved.

Group Morale

Morale represents a feeling of worth in belonging to a group. Morale facilitates solidarity and group identification necessary for successful group participation.

The morale of the group depends upon the personal involvement and identification of the group's norms. The greater the norms shared, and the more one believes in them, the more involved its members will be.

The experienced leader or activity director will notice that the sharing of departmental and agency goals and the identification of values and norms of the staff will enhance morale and group cohesiveness. Thus, group cohesiveness, group norms and group morale will act as a catalyst to increase group productivity.

Types of Groups

Through the research and study of groups, social scientists have been able to identify a variety of groups. The literature indicates certain characteristics or patterns which help classify groups. Shivers identifies three types of groups: "The primal, the mutually consensual, and the deliberately Organized."[13]

The Primal Group

This is the most deeply rooted involuntary group and is also known as the family. It offers lifetime membership. The group is homogeneous although its members may have traits originating from a variety of religious, educational, political or social backgrounds. This group seems to be at the root of society and provides the foundation for societal growth.

The Mutual Consent Group

This informal group is usually voluntary in origin and offers its members a certain pleasurable experience through interpersonal relationships. Such groups include social groups or friendships. These groups do not have strong internal structures and are vulnerable to outside pressures and forces.

The Deliberately Organized Group

This group has been deliberately formed to help achieve a specific goal. This group usually has a specific aim and philosophy and maintains a formal structure. Its objectives are reached through the assigned duties of its members whose responsibilities help achieve group unity. This type of group often forms because its members share a common belief and therefore are able to obtain their objectives in a collective fashion. Such a group may include the resident council of a nursing home.

A knowledge of group dynamics will help provide the recreation leader with a basis of knowledge necessary for organizing, implementing and conducting his own group programs. Without the ability of the recreation leader to lead and guide his group, the value of the recreation experience will certainly be diminished.

QUALITIES AND TRAITS OF THE RECREATION LEADER

As previously discussed, the literature suggests that leaders do not evolve solely as a result of specific characteristics. On the other hand, several studies and theorists do suggest that certain traits are necessary for leadership development. These include:

Intelligence

It seems logical that anyone in a leadership position will possess the intelligence required to assume the responsibilities of his position. This intelligence will enable the leader to perform his duties, which include the ability to solve problems and communicate effectively with group members.

Sensitivity

Sensitivity evolves from traits such as warmth, patience, empathy and sympathy. These traits facilitate good interpersonal relations and the ability to understand and manage others. The very nature of the disabled elderly population necessitates sensitivity on the part of those who work with them.

Judgement

Moral standards are important in maintaining the professional philosophy of therapeutic recreation both for an activity director and an activity leader. Good judgement and a sense of personal responsibility will allow the recreation leader to promote the true principles of the therapeutic recreation process and its philosophy.

Integrity and Loyalty

The recreation leader must remain loyal, not only to the recreation profession and its philosophies and ideologies, but also to the goals and standards of the agency in which he works. His intelligence will allow the recreation leader to be truthful and fair, displaying loyalty and integrity to his principles.

Dependability

The recreation leader or activity director must be dependable. His dependability will be a direct measure of how well he achieves his duties. Responsibility in carrying out his duties as a leader is equally important. Those who carry out their duties with a high sense of responsibility create a feeling of security for those around them.

Creativity and Imagination

The ability to provide leadership with creativity and imagination will foster and embellish the growth and maturity of the group. Creativity will also stimulate enthusiasm among staff and/or residents.

Adaptability and Flexibility

People and situations change. The recreation leader must be flexible and able to adapt, grow and change with respect to new professional techniques and attitudes or the changing goals of his agency. The varying degrees in the physical and or psychological limitations of the nursing home population require the flexibility of the recreation leader in his approach to activity implementation.

Motivation and Desire

The recreation leader must be motivated to work diligently and energetically to carry out the goals of his profession. The nature of recreation requires the recreation leader to work extra hours, often on weekends or holidays. This type of job requires a special dedication and ambition on the part of the recreation worker.

Physical Appearance

Appearance is important in any profession, especially when working with people. Clothing should be neat and clean and appropriate. Unfortunately, may people are often judged by their appearance. An excellent recreation leader who appears sloppy and unkempt to those who don't know him will probably be seen in a negative manner. On the other hand, those who are dressed appropriatetly and present themselves well will probably be more eagerly accepted.

Many facilities ask the staff to wear uniforms. Views regarding uniforms vary. Some believe that white jackets enhance recreation services by being viewed as more professional, whereas others see uniforms as an extension of institutional oppression. Whatever the case may be, all recreation personnel should present themselves as professionals who take pride in their appearance, their clients and their profession.

PRINCIPLES AND METHODS OF LEADERSHIP

In Chapter Three we discussed the need for developing a philosophy and a goal. Keeping in mind that therapeutic recreation aims toward the achievement of increased functional behavior, we must always have a goal.

The leader is the person primarily responsible for moving and directing his group toward the achievement of his goal. Enthusiastic and creative leadership will stimulate group members into moving with the leader toward goal achievement. An understanding of the group members' needs will also help in creating mutual satisfaction and, finally, goal achievement. Thus, it is the responsibility of the leader to keep the group moving until its goals are reached.

Teaching and Learning

Goal achievement will be accomplished in part by the ability of the leader to teach or instruct the group member or his client effectively. The leader should be aware of certain principles or concepts to be utilized with the teaching process.

Individual Assessment

It is important for the leader to assess his client regarding his ability and learning pace. Individual differences must be considered so that instruction will be attainable for each client. "Graded activity levels" can be used to categorize "low," "medium," or "high" functioning residents. Thus, consideration of physical and or psychological limitations and their influence upon individual learning capabilities are essential for each client. Asking an elderly resident who can't read to participate in the drama group would not be a good starting point for that resident. Thus, learning abilities as well as the resident's social, educational or cultural background will certainly influence the teaching process of the recreation leader.

A Supportive Environment

It is especially important for the elderly to know that they can still learn. A supportive environment in a noncompetitive atmosphere will increase positive responses or performances. Studies have shown that elderly individuals whose performances were being "evaluated" or "compared" to others usually did worse than those placed in a supportive, non-threatening situation.[14]

Within a noncompetitive atmosphere it is also important to provide the elderly with positive reinforcement of learned tasks. The elderly resident learning a folk dance needs immediate, positive reinforcement to help encourage correct responses. Reinforcements and encouragement are important teaching tools.

"Hands on" Learning

Involving the client in an active role or "hands on" situation will act as a catalyst to the learning process. Teaching nursing home residents to folk dance will probably have little success without the resident actually doing the dance.

Practice

The old adage "Practice makes perfect" is an important catalyst in the learning process. Any human being, regardless of age, requires the opportunity to practice what he has learned. Practicing skills of the elderly as activities will increase their performance levels. Rehearsals or practice sessions with the elderly in activities such as drama groups or choral groups are essential to the success of the activity and the ability of the residents to learn the required material.

THE ROLE OF THE RECREATION LEADER

An understanding of leadership theories, methods, techniques and styles will certainly help provide the recreation leader with a solid foundation of group dynamics. However, understanding these theories without the ability to translate them into leadership practices will certainly affect his performance as an effective leader.

Educational Background

Our struggles to gain status as an occupation and profession must continue on every level. Directly related to the high quality service we deliver is the need for recreation leaders with an adequate and appropriate educational background. The recreation leader should be a person who has earned a degree in recreational service from an accredted facility.

A sound academic education will help provide the recreation leader with a philosophy and rationale upon which he can deliver a sound system of therapeutic recreation services.

Responsibilities of the Recreation Leader

The development of a well balanced recreation program will enable the recreation leader to carry out his duties and perform his job responsibilities to the fullest extent possible.

We have discussed the general role of the effective leader earlier in this chapter. The following list delineates the wide variety of duties and responsibilities of the recreation leader in the long-term care facility. All of these responsibilities are carried out under the supervision and direction of the department supervisor or director.

The Recreation Leader:

1. Works directly with his client, planning implementing and conducting a variety of recreation activities for the active and passive client.

2. Instructs and teaches individual clients a variety of skills necessary for participation in activities.

3. Provides choices for activity participation enabling the participant to achieve a meaningful, satisfying experience.

4. In relation to #3, determines capabilities of the client and seeks to interest him in social situations. Seeks to assist in the integration of the individual with the facilities or agencies environment.

5. Encourages client participation in trips and outings.

6. Uses the agencies facilities in obtaining supplies, materials, and equipment necessary for specific activities.

7. Maintains correspondence in relation to programs.

8. Attends inter-disciplinary team conferences and team meetings related to the area for which he is assigned.

9. Supervises volunteers assigned to assist him or his area.

10. Participates in production of client newsletter.

11. Assists director in soliciting outside organizations for talent and gifts or donations.

12. Meets with client committees as requested.

13. Prepares attendance reports and activity summaries.

14. Writes client care plan and progress notes as required by the agency and regulating bodies.

15. Interviews, assesses and evaluates all newly admitted clients to the facility to which he is assigned.

16. Registers newly admitted clients to vote.

17. Attends in-service programs and related workshops.

Activity Specialists

Activity specialists are employees who have been trained and who have a specialized degree (music, art etc.) from an accredited institution. The activity specialist utilizes his technical skills, specialized training and educational background to develop and implement a comprehensive program in his area of specialization. The specialist may work with the activity leader to help augment the activities program or he may work alone with individual clients.

"Hands on" contact with the long-term care client of the recreation department emanates from the recreation leader as he conducts activity programs. The importance of hiring a professional, well educated recreation leader cannot be overemphasized. The significance of furthering our profession through every employee we hire must be stressed. Subscriptions to professional literature and organizations, attendance at workshops and conferences and the understanding of human and group dynamics will enhance the professional background of the recreation leader.

The Role of the Supervisor or Director

The role of the supervisor will have a significant effect upon the success of the recreation program and the entire department. The most well equipped, well staffed recreation department will probably have little success without a competent and qualified supervisor to lead and direct it in carrying out its administrative duties and achieving departmental goals.

Supervision goes beyond personnel management. Effective supervision should include employee growth, client satisfaction and program organization and development.[15] It should include innovative and creative recreation services to the maximum number of clients possible.

Long-term care facilities vary in size and administrative policy. Certain facilities employ a recreation director who also acts as department supervisor, while other facilities may employ a director and supervisor.

Whatever the supervisory responsibilities may be, it is the role of the director or supervisor to accomplish his duties through achieving the goals of both his department and agency. The following list delineates the responsibilities and functions of the recreation director or supervisor.

The director is responsible for:

1. The department of recreation which conducts a seven day a week series of varied social, cultural, recreational, educational and religious activities.
2. Planning and budgeting for and execution of activities program.

3. The promulgation of departmental policies and the inter-
    pretation of such policies to his staff in order to carry out
    programming and effectively accomplish departmental
    goals.

4. Interpreting recreation and agency goals to outside organ-
    izations and professionals for purposes of program en-
    hancement and public relations.

5. Exercising leadership and direction to staff regarding plan-
    ning, implementation and execution of activity programs.

6. Employment and termination of departmental staff.

7. Offering guidance toward professional growth, evaluation
    of work performance and stimulating their loyalty and
    dedication to the field.

8. Providing open lines of communication through informal
    channels as well as through staff meetings and individu-
    alized staff conferences and supervisory meetings. Meetings
    should include evaluations of worker's abilities and meth-
    ods of activity programming.

9. Providing continuing education programs and professional
    conferences and workshops to all staff.

10. Working with committees of residents to further interests
    of client population and improve the program.

11. Relating to the administration and or board of trustees, in-
    terpreting agency goals to staff as well as staff needs and
    concerns to administration.

12. Coordinating transportation and insurance for outings.

13. Overseeing publication of client newspaper.

14. Overseeing functioning of client library.

15. Supervising volunteers and fieldwork students assigned
    from local colleges and universities.

Factors for Effective Supervision

Every supervisor or director carries out his job duties in a manner indicative of his own individual personality and professional style. Regardless
of style, effective leadership becomes easier to accomplish when it is based
upon the principles of democracy. A primary objective of the activity director
is satisfying the program and agency needs while maintaining sensitivity
toward the needs of his employees.

An effective supervisor accomplishes departmental goals through creating an atmosphere conducive to a cooperative effort. An environment

which facilitiates high morale will stimulate the employee's desire to carry out his job more effectively.

The following factors need to be considered for effective supervision:

1. A feeling of mutual trust and respect should be created. The supervisor must exhibit a feeling of confidence and trust among his staff.

2. Work assignments and delegations of jub duties should be distributed equally. In relation to this, the effective supervisor will need to review periodically the required work load and ensure that needed adjustments are made to meet goals on time.

3. Creativity among workers needs to be stimulated by the supervisor. An ability to develop new and creative ideas, formulating them to meet the needs of the facility is essential. All staff should have the opportunity to contribute suggestions, ideas and in-put regarding departmental policy and program enhancement.

4. The supervisor must maintain a satisfactory level of departmental morale. He must be fair and impartial to employees. A sincere interest and a supportive attitude toward the staff will result in staff cooperation and trust.

5. Evaluation and conferences are essential. Constructive guidance, individual supervision and one to one contact are necessary in fostering a supportive and caring environment for the staff.

6. Flexibility is essential. The issue of time needs flexibility on the part of the supervisor. The nature of recreation requires work at odd hours, evenings, holidays and weekends. The supervisor who overlooks the *occasional* latecomer will receive more from the staff in the end. Penny-pinching with time does not lead to cooperative efforts by the staff.

7. All staff must be recognized for their skills and capabilities on a regular basis. A simple "thank you" when distributing paychecks will go a long way. Recognition for good work will inspire enthusiasm and cooperation.

8. An open line for communication is essential. The staff must be made to feel free *at any time* to communicate *any* problems or concerns (no matter how trite they may seem to be) to the supervisor. Problems cannot be solved if the supervisor is not aware of them.

9. Body language is a part of communication. The supervisor

who conveys unhappiness or concern without being explicit will create confusion and tension.

10. Silence may sometimes be the best kind of communication. The supervisor as an effective leader learns to *listen* to his staff *before* responding. Staff should be given the opportunity of communicating their idea, suggestion or problem without interruption.

The effective supervisor needs to consider factors related to those other than immediate staff. These include:

1. The ability to interface and communicate effectively with employees, administration, board of trustees, or the clients of the facility in both written and verbal forms.

2. The effective supervisor or director must be able to represent the department in dealing with outside agencies, consumers, employee groups, unions and the general public.

SUMMARY

The combination of ingredients necessary to the implementation and operation of a successful program will be of little value without effective leadership.

The program planner or activity director must have a clear understanding of the meaning of leadership and its effects upon programming and client responses. Concomitant to the understanding of leadership should be an awareness of leadership theories and styles and their appropriate utilization as related to the delivery of therapeutic recreation services.

A knowledge of human behavior, its interpersonal relationships and group dynamics is also necessary for the activity director in planning for activities for a specific client population.

Finally, the qualities and traits of leaders at all levels within the recreation department should be identified. Leadership roles, responsibilities and duties at the different levels also need to be recognized.

Regardless of the style with which leadership is carried out, certain elements distinguish effective from noneffective leaders. The effective supervisor earns respect not only for himself but for the the entire staff through creating an environment conducive to the principles of democracy.

The ship whose sails are guided by a leader with a clear destination, will create harmony and cooperation among its crew and staff, instilling in them the willingness to keep the ship afloat!

Chapter 8

RECREATION FOR THE COGNITIVELY IMPAIRED[1]

For residents with cognitive impairments, recreation can be a particularly effective form of intervention. Because of the play element associated with it, recreation presents less threat than many of the more clinically oriented treatment models. The nonthreatening atmosphere of recreation encourages freedom and relaxation, thereby mitigating the tension and anxiety experienced by older persons who suffer from impairments of judgement and memory.

While it is difficult to make an accurate assessment of the number of older persons suffering from dementing illnesses, it seems clear that the incidence of such illnesses rises with advancing age.[2] In the light of recent demographic data, the magnitude of the susceptible elderly population is, therefore, quite startling. Those over 85 years make up the most rapidly-growing segment of the American population, a group which Roth projects will reach at least 3.3 million by the year 2000, possibly even as much as 6.7 million.[3]

Probably the best known among the dementing illnesses of the elderly is Alzheimer's disease, which is characterized by progressive loss of memory, disorientation, confusion, impairment of judgment, behavioral problems and mood changes. Reports indicate that approximately 4 million Americans suffer from this disease which affects not only the elderly but, in some instances, those in late middle age.[4] Other illnesses accompanied by cognitive impairment affect some 10–20 percent of Americans over the age of 65.[5]

Alzheimer's disease has been the subject of several media presentations lately, having been identified as the most important disease of the eighties.

Earlier, the diagnosis "organic brain syndrome" was generally used to identify dementing illnesses. In popular language the word "senility" is often used to refer to any and every type of cognitive impairment, from simple slips of memory to serious deficits of judgment. The American public, including many professionals in nursing homes, tends to believe that "senility" is an inevitable accompaniment of old age.

Such expectations serve to promote the myth that cognitive impairment is a usual condition of later life. But research indicates that out of any ten persons over the age of sixty-five with signs of dementing illness, approximately five will be diagnosed with Alzheimer's disease, with two or three suffering from multi-infarct dementia (MID), and the remaining two or three identifiable as victims of other conditions affecting cognitive functioning.[6] Many of these other conditions are reversible, resulting from fevers, cardiovascular problems, metabolic disorders, reactions to medication, changes in nutritional status, and emotional problems such as depression, anxiety or boredom. Any of these conditions may affect, even seriously, the mental functioning of older adults. But, while such conditions are reversible, multi-infarct dementia, like Alzheimer's disease, is not reversible. (MID involves a series of small strokes which destroy sections of brain tissue and thus cause dementia.)

Many theories have been proposed to explain the cause of dementing illnesses in the elderly. Research on the chemistry of the aging brain has found a precipitous loss of the enzyme choline acetyltransferase in those diagnosed as having Alzheimer's disease.[7] Other studies have focused on the presence of excessive quantities of toxic elements (e.g. aluminum).[8] Further investigative theories have suggested that dementing illnesses are caused by slow-acting transmittable viruses, by failures of the immune system in later life, or by genetic factors.[9]

While such research continues to clarify the background of dementing illnesses among the elderly, much more remains to be done before successful treatments are available. In the meantime, the elderly who suffer from dementing illnesses need maximal responsive care. Although it is not yet possible to cure such patients, there are procedures available which can help them and their caregivers to cope with changes brought about by the disease. Secondary conditions related to the disease, as well as a host of individual reactions to the disease, are all frequently confused with the disease itself, and viewed as equally beyond cure. But this is not the case. While nothing can be done at present to cure the illness, these related elements can definitely be addressed.

Reactive response to illness is, of course, a general and wide-ranging phenomenon, but illnesses that reduce mental competence produce particularly strong reactions. On the broadest level, societal response to dementing illness combines fear, withdrawal, and even contempt. Older adults who regarded themselves (and have been regarded by society) as perfectly normal, and who discover evidence of mental "slippage" are un-derstandably terrified at the possibility of passing into the category of the demented. Initial memory lapses bring the victim gradually to a realization that something is awry with his cognitive processes, that elemental controls are slipping.

Reactions to this realization can be as pernicious in their effects as the disease itself, producing frenzy, deepening depression, helplessness, even despair. Among primary caregivers, whether relatives at home or staff in the nursing home, response can likewise be severe, ranging from helpless incomprehension to resentment and rage. Stages of denial, anger, and depression are easliy discernable in those whose spouses, parents or close friends gradually exhibit undeniable symptoms of dementing illness.[10]

Because such illness is usually characterized by insidious onset, the early stages are vague and hard to define, with initial symptomatic behavior excused as trivial and as mere momentary lapse or misunderstanding. Gradually, however, spouses and other family members must take up more and more "behavioral slack" to sustain the individual suffering from de-menting illness. Faced with this undeniable evidence of failing competency, both victim and caretaker begin to experience the range of reactive responses mentioned above. As the demands of daily maintenance become more and more consuming, and the reactions to the illness exact their toll on both victim and family, a point is eventually reached where care can no longer be continued at home and families, with deep regret, must place their loved ones in long-term care institutions.

But institutional placement, by itself, does not guarantee that disease-related reactions will be adequately recognized or treated. For the most part the elderly with dementing illnesses do not receive special provision in treatment plans. Carl Eisdorfer, calling for increased programs for these patients, laments the fact that many professionals do not consider them capable of rehabilitation.[11] Because of such appraisals, programs for the elderly with cognitive impairments are often poorly planned, or not planned at all. Generally the care provided for them is not therapeutic or rehabi-litative in aim, but simply custodial. At best it is aimed at keeping such residents from harming themselves and others, at worst, it is aimed at keeping them out of the staff's way. Such care as they do receive is often left to nonprofessional attendants with little training for their difficult task, and little understanding of their patients' illnesses.

These staff members frequently "label" cognitively impaired patients in stereotypic fashion. They see them as less than normal; often they fear that the patients, in their frustration, will be hostile and even violent. Given these attitudes and the general lack of special preparation for such caregiving roles, the worker-patient relationship is liable only to aggravate the emo-tional state of the client. (This is also a painful example of how, within the long-term care structure, workers on the primary care level are lost as possible sources of patient strength, as important resources for preserving patient self-esteem.)

In the face of such individual and institutional difficulties, therapeutic recreation can offer successful intervention with elderly patients suffering from dementing illnesses. In principle, the intervention seeks to counterbalance residents' loss of self-esteem, as well as their loss of a sense of control over life. In addition, the therapeutic intervention seeks to offset staff and family judgments that residents are incapable of purposeful behavior, a judgment which, of course sets the stage for expectation-fulfilling behavior.

Reversing negative expectations calls for innovative program planning on the part of therapeutic recreation personnel. But patients with cognitive impairments have many remaining personal resources which the recreation program can tap. When residual strengths are mobilized, new skills can be acquired, the spiral of failure is broken, and the quality of life is improved, permitting hope for further gains. Thus the costs of innovative programs are more justified when program objectives and goals are met.

EFFECTIVE PROGRAMMING

An effective program requires, in the first place, a staff dedicated to the goals and objectives established for the patient group. This entails a philosophy committed to rehabilitative aims and to the working assumption that clients are capable of improvement. The importance of this underlying philosophy cannot be overemphasized. While recognizing that dementing illness cannot be reversed, the staff perceives that therapeutic recreation intervention can reverse some of the accompanying disorders, thus permitting maximum utilization of residual cognitive, affective, social and physical strengths.

Selection of staff to work with this client group is obviously important. Only those staff members who are able to offer what Rogers describes as total positive regard can really affirm the strengths of the cognitively impaired.[12] Enormous patience is required to deal with shifts in mood and in level of skill. All members of the staff team, both professional and paraprofessional, will need intensive and on-going training. Since their work is so demanding, they may especially profit from opportunities to discuss and work through the emotional aspects of their service.

SPECIAL CONSIDERATIONS FOR THE ALZHEIMER'S PATIENT

Within long-term care facilities, residents with dementing illnesses are usually separated from those whose cognitive functioning is intact.[13] While there are arguments for and against such segregation, it does facilitate the creation of programs especially designed for the cognitively impaired; it also spares these patients from having to compete with others in a common recreation setting. Whether physically separated or not, these programs will, of course, require some special adaptations. A major factor to consider is the tendency of Alzheimer's patients to wander. (Indeed, some research has sought to measure the efficacy of specific recreation programs reducing wandering behavior).[14] In this regard, Panella and McDowell have found that disquising entrances helps prevent wandering.[15] They also suggest that a single large room divided by moveable partitions affords the most useful program space. As these authors note, patients with dementing illnesses are especially sensitive to the physical environment, and require a setting which is neither too large nor too small.

Safety is of particular importance in working with residents whose cognitive impairments may prevent them from recognizing objects in their environment, even objects that should be somewhat familiar to them. Thus, they may trip over a quite visible protruding piece of furniture, or they may be frightened by a colored pattern in the linoleum, which they perceive as potentially dangerous. Glare on surfaces may alarm or confuse them. It is not difficult to imagine how frightening ordinary things can be for them, since, simply put, these residents can no longer interpret the messages which they receive from their ordinary sensory intake.

Readily accessible bathrooms are required, and floor coverings which can easily be cleaned are the most practical. Although toilet training programs can sometimes be very helpful with these patients, at other times, especially as the disease progresses, they do not succeed. It is helpful also to remember that these residents are easily distracted. Therefore it is wise to keep bathrooms free of adornment, especially mirrors, which can prove to be particularly absorbing to patients who are past the earlier stages of their illness.

ACTIVITIES FOR THE ALZHEIMER PATIENT

Although older persons with dementing illness are often viewed as incapable of participating in or enjoying recreational activities, there are many programs which can prove rewarding to such patients. Since their cognitive functioning is impaired, it is important that the tasks involved in a particular recreational activity do not excel their skill level. It is equally important (though often overlooked in program planning) that activities do not simply call for tasks *below* their skill level. Further careful assessment of program content is required by the fact that the cognitive impairments of residents vary greatly, not only from person to person, but from time to time for the same person.

This variation is one of the most taxing and challenging elements in planning therapeutic recreation. While balancing this changing, and rather unpredicatable, level of functioning, the TR program planner must also manage to provide a fairly stable schedule. Stability of structure is especially important to this client group precisely because they have so little ability to structure their own behavior. Balancing overall programming as well as individual participation calls for great sensitivity on the part of the recreation professional. In essence the task is one requiring masterful and sensitive paradox: constant adjustment and adaptation within a fixed and stabilizing framework.

One component which is often neglected in programming for these clients is the specifically cognitive. The neglect of cognitive activities reflects, in part, the sterotypic belief that clients with impaired mentation are not capable of participating in activities with a strong cognitive element. Partly, too, the staff may feel ill at ease about the precise nature of the cognitive impairment. In the same way that some professionals may refuse to deal with the approaching death of terminally ill patients, others may find it difficult to focus on dementing illness, to address its precise limits, its demanding implications for program design.

An example of this stereotyping of cognitive inability is discussed by Phillips[16] who found that medical doctors and psychologists did not believe that residents with poor scores on the Katzman[17] indicator could participate at all in anagram-solving puzzles. Not only did Phillips find them able to participate, but he found their performance improved with cueing. Moreover, many of them commented on the pleasure it gave them to succeed at these cognitive activities. It is true, as Eisdorfer points out, that we have no evidence to suggest that such experiences have long-term effects for the cognitively-impaired elderly, but at least for the moment, the feeling of success can give a boost to their sense of self esteem.[18]

Word Games

Phillips' study, supported by others gives strong credibility and encouragement to the use of word games and word puzzles in programs for Alzheimer patients.[19] Such activities can stimulate residual problem-solving resources and may slow intellectual decline. Much more research is needed to shed light on the cognitive impact of activities of this sort. But such research is difficult to conduct, because of the careful proection of the rights of these patients.[20] Professional and institutional safeguards for incompetent clients, especially in terms of research, have become quite restrictive in recent years. In addition, relatives or other advocates frequently refuse permission for participation in such research, often out of a mix of protective motives and an assumption that such clients could not cognitively manage the requirements of the research. Unfortunately, without good, solid research dependable information about the recreation behavior and cognitive capacities of these elderly will continue to be sparse.

In terms of constructing actual programs, designing an anagram-solving activity or other word game for the cognitively impaired is not essentially different from preparing such an activity for any group of adults. What is different is client assessment—the level of functioning is liable to be much more changeable and unpredictable, and the pace, too, may have to be much slower than for general clients. Creative writing is another form of activity which is primarily cognitive in content, but which draws upon the rich affective resources of the client. It is vitally important that these resources not be disregarded in the face of decreasing cognitive ability. In fact, there is no evidence to suggest that affectivity is diminished—the intense rage and deep despair observed in these clients, attest to the strength of their emotional resources. They require an outlet, one which can be meaningful, productive and rewarding.

Creative Writing

Creative writing can afford such an outlet, and since it so closely allies cognitive and affective functioning, it is particularly appropriate as a program for clients with impaired mentation. In implementing creative writing programs, the therapeutic recreation professional needs to carefully assess the client for any shifts in mood or sudden lessening of focus. There are prime times in each day for most people. Cognitiviely impaired elderly have these same rhythms, too. The high times, brief though they may be, are especially apt for enjoyment of creative writing. In some cases, this writing can take the form of guided fantasy. Some therapists prefer to conduct this activity in small groups, others find that the client requires almost a one-to-one relationship to profit from the activity. At times the creative writing can take the form of a journal, one that looks into a person's past experience, or one that takes the form of an imaginary conversation with an admired hero/heroine. (Respect for the client's privacy is paramount, so that only when he chooses to share the journal can the TR professional feel free to examine it.)

The purpose of writing activity is not to provide grist for psychoanalytic interpretations, but to afford opportunity for self expression. A visual image may be used to trigger response. Some therapists use outlandish or seemingly frivolous themes in order to facilitate the expression of very profound thoughts. At times it is necessary to transcribe the writing, since some clients cannot deal with written language. Other TR professionals have found a value in the physical act of writing, almost as though that behavior itself acts as a stimulant. For those who do not seem to enjoy expressive writing of this sort, communicative writing may work better. Short notes on cards at holiday times or special occasions not only help to focus on others but may also bring the reward of a response, if some family member will address and mail the cards. The notes serve, too, to reinforce reality orientation, reminding the writers of the season, its symbols and meaning.

Poetry

One very special type of creative writing is poetry. When institutional separation severs the resident's sense of past, present and future, poetry can serve as a helpful thread of continuity through time. Residents, even those who seem to be quite impaired, can be part of a poetry group, and can contribute to a collective poem, exchanging feedback with peers, and deriving from the experience not only a sense of mastery, but also a sense of belonging and sharing. By writing a poem and presenting it to others, skills and interests are revived, identity is reinforced, and past achievements are recalled.

Sharing poetry can also foster communication, for poetry deals in affect. Perception of the feelings expressed in poetry can uncover emotions and experiences long lost because of the failing memory which plagues the cognitively impaired. The act of creation, in itself, is an assertive action, which helps reinforce the concept that avenues of assertion and expression are still open. Competence and mastery have a cumulative effect here, building upon repeated successful interactions with the environment.

When any human being is cut off from adequate stimuli, from sources of information and opportunity to interact, previously attained competence levels begin to disintegrate. Again, it must be stressed that we have no evidence which suggests that the cognitively impaired elderly person can retain the impression of this moment of enjoyment and success. Perhaps the experience is totally transitory for them. It can be recalled by staff and family, however, and so for them it counters the reactive discouragement which dementing illness can so easily create. For staff and family it is also important that hope be maintained, not necessarily hope for a cure, but hope for some relief from the relentless negative experiences which the clients endure. It might be argued, although again without scientific evidence, that one's body registers the happy moments as well as the sad and frustrating ones, and this registering might have some cumulative effects on those who suffer dementing decline.[21]

Art As Activity

One activity which draws on the immense inner resources of all participants is art. In many instances, however, the task of getting a client population involved in art is difficult because they are blocked by deeply engrained attitudinal barriers. Like mathematics, art is declared off-limits for many people at a very early age. But, here, there is a distinct advantage in working with the cognitively impaired. Memory failure can actually free them from many pre-conceived notions of this sort.

An enormous value in art is its power to touch and loosen human emotions. Psychologists have long recognized the therapeutic value of the visual arts. Jung, in particular, saw artistic expression as mirroring the inner self.[22] It is important that the recreator respond sensitively to this revelation, that he acknowledge the privacy, in a sense, the sacredness, of the artistic statement. If a client volunteers to share the meaning of his work, that is a gift, not something to be taken for granted. It is also a demanding gift, for not everything revealed this way is cheering. Nevertheless, these experiences are vitally important for the cognitively impaired. Their rich emotional energies have so few outlets, and the dynamic possibilities of line and shape, of color and tone, image and abstraction, afford them a much-needed opportunity.

Nadeau recommends being generous with supplies and giving large pieces of paper, so that even the timid can have a sense of spaciousness, something perhaps particularly important for the institutionalized.[23] Experienced staff members know how carefully observant they need to be as clients work with these materials. It is important, however, that carefulness not slide into control. To avoid this, the activity leader should function essentially as a facilitator in the art session, not as a teacher. To correct or direct the art work would be to invade the creative inner space of the participating residents.

As happens with other activities described in this chapter, some of the clients hesitate to join in. Sitting on the sidelines, they may watch for several sessions before deciding to participate. Once they do, they may become the most enthusiastic members in the group. Elaine Streitfeld, Art Therapist in the Recreation Department of the Hebrew Home and Hospital for Aged, Riverdale, New York, has had exceptional success in working with Alzheimer patients.[24] Many of her clients have had one man/woman shows. She describes their delight as their paintings unfold, their satisfaction at beholding their creations, their pride as others recognize their achievement.

A number of different approaches have been suggested for helping clients get started with their painting. Nadeau describes reading a fairy tale to the group in order to trigger their imaginations.[25] Alternatively, the art group related to a reminiscence group, with the remembered material serving as the basis for creative endeavor. A very powerful stimulus can also come from using music as a background to the art session. Ingmar Bergman, the renowned Swedish movie director, has reflected on this.[26] Given the grace of his visual imagery and his powerful use of music, Bergman is compelling when he says that music touches directly on the emotions without having to pass through cognitive processes.

Arieti goes further in describing a particular kind of cognition, "amorphous cognition," which he sees related to music in a special way.[27] Described by some authors as primary process, by others as pre-conscious cognition, the product of amorphous cognition is the endocept, which in our technological society is largely suppressed or repressed in adults. Arieti's suggestion is that music permits one to be in touch with the endoceptual content. Perhaps for that reason, music is one of the most powerful activities for clients with impaired mentation, whose endoceptual content may be cognitively more significant precisely because of the limitations on other cognitive functioning.

Musical Programs

Therapeutic Recreation professionals have long recognized the strength of musical programs for every population. Poignant stories from the recreation literature attest to the effectiveness of music in drawing out the isolate, cheering the depressed, and uniting the disparate. In this regard, music programs for the cognitively impaired do not differ dramatically from those for other adults. What difference there is lies not so much in the programming process, as in the particular significance music holds for these clients.

Not only is music a pleasurable mode of expression for them, but since it continues within their range of competence, it also represents an achievement. Music from the past has the added advantage of being familiar; for people whose memory decline keeps them in a world where most things are strange, the familiar can be very reassuring. Singing together in a group provides a sense of belonging, of sharing, of collaboration. There is, too, a sense of transcendence inherent in music, which carries one out beyond the boundaries of the self, into a larger world of meaning. A certain kind of memory is tapped in music, one more closely related to the endoceptual process. These benefits, among others, characterize music as particularly valuable for the cognitively impaired elderly.

Music programs can be designed in many ways: paired with movement, which seems to reduce wandering behavior:[28] paired with art or creative writing to increase the affective response:[29] or presented alone. Whatever the format, the musical experience, both for the performer and listener includes a complex psychological reaction to the emotional and sensory-motor stimuli, and "an awareness of the shaping logic that is unfolding the design of the composition."[30] Such awareness is necessarily present for the cognitively impaired as for any other participants, but in both cases, the awareness can occur at the level of primary, endoceptual process. Thus, while it may appear to be a passive process of listening, music-listening can indeed be very active. Just as, in certain counseling approaches, active listening is a form of communication, so too it is here.

SUMMARY

All the varied activities described in this chapter are, in essence, assertive forms of recreation, forms which permit, even elicit, an active role for the cognitively impaired participant. In some cases the assertion is more explicit than in others. Admittedly, the active role is not always recognized as appropriate for adults with diminished mentation. But research in this area is still in its very early stages. Consequently, therapeutic recreation has a unique contribution to make in developing insights into the potential of those suffering from dementing illness. It is professionally crucial that recreational therapy not create its own inner obstacles to this investigation by supporting stereotypes and allowing primitive labeling of the impaired elderly. These residents are capable of much more than we facilely imagine and assiduously expect. We limit them by our own doubts and dark expectations.

Our technological society highly values mature cognition, that secondary mental process which involves categories, figures, facts, and manipulation of empirical data. But much of the wealth of human experience occurs at the primary level, the level of the creative arts. Recreation is one area where the primary processes can be pursued, and for that reason therapeutic recreation may be seen as the treatment of choice for the cognitively impaired elderly. To be at leisure, to be free, even from conceptual restraints, is the ultimate goal of many spiritual ideologies. Some of the cognitive shackles which spiritual people spend years trying to shed are already removed from the person with impaired mentation. One might argue then, that such persons are in an advantageous position for pursuing true leisure, that their capacity for pure play is greater than that of most people because their limiting condition has, strangely, freed them.

On the other hand, it must be admitted that at times recreation professionals mistakenly reduce play to an infantalizing form. But in the psychological dynamics of someone like Eric Berne for example, the child in us actually represents a high degree of freedom—just the opposite of a childish regression to dependency and pre-mature activity.[31] Recreational activities which are regressive, which resemble busy-work given to children, will not promote feelings of growth, achievement, and self worth. On the contrary, they will only demoralize clients, family, and staff.

The recreation therapist who can have faith in the hidden potential of the cognitively impaired, will be more than pleasantly surprised; he will be overwhelmed and left with moments of wonder. When Elaine Streitfeld, quoted above, organized art sessions for Alzheimer patients in a large New York nursing home, she originally expected that through this activity she would help residents escape from their unpleasant, confining world.[32] She found just the opposite: they took her into their inner world, and she was astonished at the wealth she found there.

Again and again, those who have kept faith with this very special group of clients have discovered, in the poignant marks of their illness, distress that harbored mystery, pain and endurance that spoke courage, loss and poverty that kept spirit. Such experiences tell us that we are not facilely beyond or above those who suffer dementing illness. Indeed, they trace out elemental truths about all human capacity and power, all human vulnerability and need. Seeing *our* human lot writ in their condition can only clarify the large claim they have on us.

Chapter 9

THE UTILIZATION OF VOLUNTEER SERVICES

THE DEVELOPMENT OF VOLUNTEER SERVICES

The motivating force behind the development of volunteer services can be traced to the various health fields, particularly the hospital setting.

Within the medical setting, the role of the volunteer was to offer good cheer and visit with the sick. However, as the role and function of the hospital changed so, too, did the needs of its community.

Changes in the entire concept of the health care field resulted in the establishment of nursing homes, geriatric day centers, community centers and adult homes. These changes lead to the alteration and expansion of volunteer services from custodial care to the treatment of the "total human being." These services included all aspects of the hospital and nursing home setting such as recreation, social service, dietary and nursing.[1]

Since the American Nursing Home Association sparked the establishment of the Volunteer and Activity Service Corps in 1968, community volunteers have successfully provided services dramatically affecting rehabilitation programs in the hospital and nursing home setting.[2]

The expansion of volunteerism also comes with the increased leisure time of American citizens. Mandatory retirement and more sophisticated patterns of leisure lifestyles has added significantly to the use of volunteers as a human resource.

The development of volunteer programs as an organized structure and delivery service brought new concerns which required attention. Program standards, professional preparation and responsibility for the administration of such programs needed to be addressed.

ADMINISTRATIVE SANCTIONS

As discussed previously, it is of primary importance for the administration to set the tone which creates a milieu necessary to the well being of every resident or patient of the nursing home or hospital.

It is his responsibility to create an environment which also regards the utilization of volunteer services as essential to the patient's well being. Further, he must be able to translate the meaning of volunteer services as a significant contribution to all departments and their staff.

The volunteer department must not be construed as a service area which deserves less than other any other discipline. Administrative support must be concommitant with the needs of the department, including a director, a secretary, supplies and a realistic budget.

THE MEANING AND VALUE OF VOLUNTEERISM

The value of volunteer services is apparent in its contribution to the patient's well being. In addition to providing one's talent and time, the volunteer offers the patient the security of knowing that he is being remembered.

The contribution of the volunteer extends beyond the scope of comforting the patient. Volunteers often provide services which complement staff talent or expertise and may significantly add to the efficient operation of a particular department.

The volunteers' services may also be seen as contributing to the entire welfare of the nursing home and its community.[3] Through their experience they help explode the myths of aging, thereby communicating to others the true value of the institutionalized aged.

Finally, the value of volunteering is the satisfaction of one's own personal need and gratification as a worthwhile human being. The feeling of helping those less fortunate is certainly a motivating factor in helping oneself feel better.

The increased amount of leisure time as well as mandatory retirement ages may also be a precipitating factor of increased volunteer services. The need to fill one's time with a worthwhile leisure activity is becoming easier to do with more time available. Volunteering may help fill the time for those whose families have grown and whose visits are now less frequent. Finally, the person who feels better about himself will be considered a citizen who contributes to the democratic ideals of the community and society at large.

With an understanding of the needs and value of volunteer services and the support of administration, a director of volunteers must be selected.

Selecting a Volunteer Director

As discussed in earlier chapters, all the elements of an activities department will be of little value without a well qualified, experienced director to lead it. The same is true of the volunteer department. Further, the hiring of a volunteer director will represent a level of importance to the department and its facility.

Although the volunteer may not have a degree specifically related to administration of volunteer services, he or she should be a qualified professional with a degree from an accredited college or university. The degree should be a concentration in recreation, psychology, administration, social work or another related field.[4]

The role of the director requires a job description as does the activity director. It is important to note that the activity director may wear two hats in certain facilities incorporating the duties of the volunteer director with those of the activity director. In such cases, the responsibility of the volunteer services should be incorporated into the job description of the activity director.

The following job description represents the significance of volunteer services in the long-term care facility. The role of the volunteer director should encompass:

1.   The planning, administration and coordination of volunteers and volunteer services in all units of the facility. This includes a knowledge of the structure and operation of the entire facility and its departments.

2.   Assisting the agency in the delivery of care to residents by obtaining and retaining an adequate, competent and satisfied volunteer staff to augment the services of personnel.

3.   Serving as advisor to administration on the use of volunteers, trends in volunteerism, and on policies and procedures relating to the volunteer department.

Specific responsibilities include:

1.   Recruiting volunteers from the community and cooperating agencies.

2.   Utilizing of community resources for securing volunteers for special events or in emergencies.

3.   Arranging special receptions and tours of facilities for potential volunteers.

4.   Surveying volunteers' needs of institution and developing job descriptions.

5. Interpreting the role of the volunteer to staff members. It is essential that staff clearly understand that volunteers complement staff services rather than replace them. Staff should realize that effective use of volunteers result in greater care of all residents.

6. Interviewing, selection and assignment of volunteers.

7. Orientating and training of volunteers.

8. Developing continuing education programs for volunteers.

9. Evaluating of volunteers and volunteer program. Confering with department heads for volunteer appraisals.

10. Organizing of recognition programs and procedures.

11. Handling complaints and disiplinary actions for volunteers.

12. Promoting community interest in volunteer services by speaking to and consulting with civic groups and educational institutions.

13. Participating in administration planning for those programs requiring the use of volunteers.

14. Devising special programs of interest to and for residents in addition to usual staffing requirements.

15. Developing of all departmental needs, records, reports and statistics.

16. Preparing publicity materials.

17. Preparing all training manuals.

OFFICE FACILITIES

Just as the location of recreation lounges and areas are crucial to the success of the activities program, so, too, is the location of the volunteer office and its facilities.

The volunteer office needs to be located in a centralized area, providing easy access to all volunteers. Adequate space for personal belongings of volunteers is also necessary.

LEGAL CONSIDERATIONS

Legal considerations must be accounted for in providing volunteer services. In most cases, volunteers will be included in the insurance plans of the agency. However, all aspects of legal concerns should be investigated with any volunteer department. Since legalities and laws vary with every state, legal advice should be sought by every agency regarding appropriate insurance for volunteers and the services they provide.

VOLUNTEER BUDGET

The volunteer department requires an operating budget. Budgeted expenses should include:

1. Salaries of the director and secretary.
2. Mailing expenses.
3. Travel expenses.
4. Reimbursement for lunch or other meals when appropriate.
5. Expenses for speaking engagements and meetings.
6. Expenses for awards.
7. Expenses for recognition parties and ceremonies.

ADMINISTRATION OF VOLUNTEER SERVICES

Administration of volunteer services requires a variety of skills and responsibilities which include volunteer:

recruitment
selection
interviews
orientation and training
assignments
evaluation
recognition
record keeping and reports

Volunteer Recruitment

Recruitment is a crucial element to volunteer services. Several methods and places for recruitment are available.[5]

First, and probably the most effective method, is personal contact by the volunteer director who can discuss the nature, scope and duties of the volunteer being sought. The needs and benefits of both the volunteer and residents can be discussed. Personal contact also allows for questions and concerns to be raised. Telephone contact may also be utilized but is usually not as effective as personal contact.

Second, volunteer groups may be invited to the facility where the director can describe the needs of their service. Tours may also be arranged.

Third, media presentations can be utilized. Brochures or pamphlets explaining the needs of volunteers can be described. Television and radio announcements can also be used. Posters in store windows, community centers and schools may also help recruit volunteers. The public relations department of the facility (when available) may also help arrange media coverage and advertisements. However, one should caution that the use of media and mass advertisements can create certain problems. Mass media may lead to an overabundance of volunteers who may not be needed. Further, certain volunteers who respond may not be appropriate.

Finally, utilization of the volunteer himself may help to spread the word when other volunteers are needed. A satisfied volunteer may help recruit through his own enthusiasm for helping others.

Recruitment of volunteers requires the knowledge of community organizations and volunteer resources. Personal contact by the director is necessary to establish a relationship between the two agencies.

Some community based organizations which may be considered a resource for volunteers are:

1. Public schools
2. Colleges and universities
3. Churches or synagogues
4. YMCAs or YMHAs
5. Senior citizen centers
6. Retired Senior Volunteer Program (RSVP)
7. Hadassah
8. ORT
9. Mayor's Office for Voluntary Action
10. Catholic or Protestant charities

Areas of Volunteer Work

Volunteer assignments vary throughout the long-term care facility. Volunteers who work directly with the patient include services such as:

Assisting with feeding and activities of daily living of residents.
Assisting with recreation activities.
Transporting of residents to clinic areas and recreation activities.
Selling candies and notions from candy carts.

Other services which do not require direct contact with residents are:

Clerical work in different departments.

Receptionist work in areas throughout the facility.

Volunteers are an essential ingredient in augmenting the services of the recreation department. Some of these services are:

Assisting at recreation activities.

Conducting recreation activities: retired teachers or professionals are often used to conduct discussion groups or classes in the area of their expertise, i.e., English classes, bingo games, music programs, etc.

Setting up and serving refreshments at activities and special events.

Transporting residents to and from activities.

Selling greeting cards and stamps.

Acting as librarians in resident library.

Showing movies.

Assisting residents in writing articles for resident publication.

Clerical work: assisting with filing, attendance statistics, typing, stapling, collating, phone messages.

Assisting with collating and stapling of activity programs.

Assisting with delivery of resident notices.

Assisting with resident outings, barbecues and garden parties.

Volunteers serve both on a regular and occasional basis. Those who serve on a regular basis can be assigned to specific duties which require continuity of services. Those who serve irregularly can be utilized for assitance with special events or occasional jobs.

Volunteer Selection

It is imperative that the volunteer director have precise knowledge regarding job assignments required by the volunteers in each department. It is therefore necessary for each department head to provide a job description to the volunteer director. This should include:[6]

A description of the required job duties and volunteer responsibilities.

Special skills required.

Approximate length of time for the job.

Days and hours of the job.

Anticipated problems on the job.

Name of supervisor for the job.

Appropriate placement depends upon adequate job descriptions.

The Interview Process

The interview process is probably the most crucial element in volunteer selection. Previous to the interview, the volunteer should complete an application which includes the applicant's name, address, age, references, occupation (former occupation if retired), specific skills and interests.

The volunteer deserves an interview equal to that of hiring a new employee. Through the interview, the volunteer director will help to create an atmosphere conducive to communication between the applicant and the director.

Throughout the interview process, the director should be gaining information necessary to determine whether or not the prospective applicant will be appropriate for the volunteer services required. Information regarding the applicant's attitude, personality and temperament, interests, skills, former background, age, etc. should be obtained. Further, the interview process should allow the volunteer to learn more about the facility and job he will be required to do.

In certain cases, volunteers may be hired for special jobs in a particular department or area. In this case, it is common for the appropriate department head to interview the applicant as well. When the volunteer is accepted, he will need to be notified regarding the time and place of training, orientation and the date work will begin. If the candidate is unacceptable, he must be told so. This is undoubtedly a difficult job. However, the reasons for rejection must be explained. Whether or not the volunteer is accepted, a completed application and notes regarding the interview process should be maintained.

Orientation and Training

It is important to distinguish between orientation and training. Orientation is the responsibility of the director in orienting the volunteer as to the environment in which he will work. Training is the responsibility of the director in whose department the volunteer is assigned. Although orientation and training must be done separately, the department heads and volunteer director must work in close harmony. Without the support of all departments heads and their participation in orientation and training sessions, the volunteer services will be unsuccessful.

Orientation sessions should be carefully planned. The following are suggested by the author and The Volunteer and Activity Corps Handbook.[7]

1. A background of the agency or nursing home and its role and place within the community it serves.
2. Agency philosophy, goals and objectives.
3. A review of the agency structure and administrative organization.
4. The overall needs of the residents including medical, nursing, social service, spiritual, religious and leisure.
5. Review of physical and/or psychological limitations of the aged population and diseases common to the elderly.
6. An overall method or approach to patient care.
7. The structure and operation of the volunteer department.
8. The general role, function and responsibility of the volunteer as he relates to the agency and volunteer director.
9. Accepted practices, policies and procedures for volunteers.
10. A tour of the facility.

Training sessions should be arranged for volunteers by the department heads of each department to which they are assigned. Training sessions should consist of:

1. Description of specific job duties of the volunteer.
2. Relationship of the volunteer to staff with the assigned department.
3. A description of departmental needs.
4. A description of department services in relation to resident needs.

Volunteer Assignments

Volunteer assignments are the responsibility of the director. The success of the volunteer department depends upon the appropriate assignment of the volunteer. Certain factors should be considered for proper volunteer assignments.[8]

1. A job description.
2. The interest of the volunteer.
3. Volunteer skills and abilities.

4. Personality of the volunteer and his supervisor.

5. The amount of supervision available for each volunteer.

Volunteer Evaluation

Evaluation of volunteers is a necessary ingredient to the success of the program. Volunteers should be evaluated by the director and the department supervisor. Some states and regulatory agencies require written evaluations of volunteers by the supervisor of the department to which they are assigned.

Further, evaluation provides feedback which results in improved performance. Evaluation of the total program is also necessary to ensure that agency needs are being met.

The Volunteer and Activity Service Corps Handbook cites some of the following questions as guides toward program evaluation.[9]

1. Were the principles and standards interpreted adequately for members of the Volunteer and Activity Service Corps?

2. Does the volunteer program have the support of the community the nursing home serves?

3. Are all community resources utilized by the volunteer program?

4. Do the activities provided by the volunteers serve the needs of the patients?

5. Are volunteers satisfied with their work, their participation, and arrangements and facilities provided them by the home?

6. Are volunteers receiving recognition?

7. Do the patients seem to benefit and enjoy the volunteer program?

8. Has the program made any noticeable changes in the attitudes and behavior of the residents?

Volunteer Awards and Recognition

Every human being needs to be recognized. The volunteer is no exception. Awards should be provided on a regular basis, at least yearly through formal recognition ceremonies. It is important for staff, administration and community representatives to attend. Certificates or pins based on the length of service are customarily provided. Other forms of recognition may include smaller, more informal teas, parties or luncheons.

Finally, many volunteers receive recognition through the satisfaction of doing their job. A comment often repeated by volunteers is: "A thank you from the resident is enough pay for me." Regardless of the type of award presented, the volunteer deserves to be recognized for contributing to the overall welfare of the resident and successful operation of the nursing home or agency.

Staff Volunteers

The increased use of nursing home staff is being recognized as an additional valuable volunteer resource. At The Jewish Home and Hospital for Aged, two new staff volunteer programs have been implemented.

A group of 50 staff members from several departments have been trained as certified feeders. Once a week, each staff volunteer helps feed a resident on a skilled nursing floor.

Another group of staff have become volunteers of the telephone support group. Each of these staff members, telephones a resident providing social interaction and emotional support to those who normally have few visitors and few social outlets.

The success of these programs have been insurmountable. The resident receives a valuable service adding to the quality of life in the nursing home. A re-assuring hand by the staff volunteer adds another dimension of security and comfort to the sometimes forgotten resident. Staff who have little resident contact (i.e. secretarys, accountants, personnel managers, etc.) provide a unique personalized service on a level they are usually not afforded. The combination of employee and volunteer provide a satisfaction, self fulfillment and reward which goes beyond the value of the pay check.

SUMMARY

As noted, the value of volunteer services has taken on special significance in the long-term care facility. Continued reassessment of budgets and staff pattern have added to the demands of volunteer services in a variety of recreation areas.

Often, the activity director plays the part of the volunteer director as well. Regardless of this, the selection of a volunteer director and the volunteer services necessitates the complete support and sanction of the administration.

It is imperative that the volunteer/activity director be qualified to interview, recruit, orient and train volunteers. An awareness regarding the required areas for volunteer work in recreation is also necessary.

Finally, the ability to offer recognition both formally and informally is required.

The successful utilization of volunteer services will be an invaluable asset to the therapeutic recreation program.

Chapter 10

THE PAPER WORK DILEMMA

DEALING WITH THE PAPER WORK DILEMMA

Dealing with the increased amount of paper work has become a challenge to activity directors everywhere.

Ideally, most activity professionals would like to provide more hours of activity programming and less staff time devoted to paper work. However, paper work *is* a necessity and this is a fact we cannot deny. As bleek as it may sometimes seem, however, there are some answers to the paper work dilemma.

Just as we continually seek new ideas and creative suggestions for activity programming, we must also seek similar solutions to the paper work dilemma. Our approach toward this challenge must be realistic; we must provide ways of accomplishing required paper work through increased staff productivity utilizing a systematized process for all areas of paper work. An organized approach (which will be described for each area of paper work) will bring more effective results using less staff time and affording more precious program hours.

The paper work process goes *beyond* the time spent writing the actual notes. Time is spent learning about residents, communicating with recreation staff and other related professionals regarding resident behaviors, problems and progress. Time is spent tracking down missing charts, finding new residents to interview or signing residents up for an outing or special event. All of these activities must be included as time related events delegated to the accomplishment of a high quality of paper work.

It is for this reason that a systematized approach incorporating all of these variables must be purposefully designed to accomplish the challenge of the paper work dilemma.

It is important to note that the activity department probably has more required paper work than the other therapy departments of the long-term care facility. Most people overlook the fact that departments such as occupational therapy and physical therapy require documentation *only* for those clients who are referred by the physician, social worker or psychiatrist and who are receiving treatment directly from their department.

The therapeutic recreation department is not afforded this luxury. Most state codes require documentation on every single resident in the facility, whether they attend activities or not. In fact, we are responsible for stating why residents are not attending and what we are doing to encourage their participation in recreation activities.

JUSTIFICATION FOR DOCUMENTATION

As difficult as it seems, there is justification for sometimes feeling overwhelmed with paper work. The following offers some rationale for paper work requirements.

Accountability as Professionals

With the struggle to obtain credibility as a profession providing services of a therapeutic nature also comes accountability for these services. One aspect of accountability lies in accurate documentation. Documentation should include areas related to:

1. Treatment care plans and progress notes.
2. Policy and procedure manuals.
3. Programming reports.
4. Progress reports to administrators.
5. Attendance records and statistics.
6. Program and staff evaluation.

Thorough, accurate records are an essential aspect of professional accountability.

Administrative Accountability and Regulatory Agencies

Accountability to administration provides another reason for accurate documentation. The rationale to administration and the board of directors for a meaningful activity program will in part be satisfied through the ability to document positive changes in resident behavior and leisure lifestyles, resulting from therapeutic recreation services.

In addition, regulatory agencies such as the State Department of Health and the Joint Commission on Accreditation of Hospitals (JCAH) require written documentation regarding the types of therapeutic recreation services being provided. Quality services are accomplished through standards set by such regulatory agencies. Documentation provides accountability to ensure that these services are in fact being met.

Staff Communication

Accurate documentation facilitates communication among staff members.[1] It is common for the activities staff to be assigned to specific areas of the facility regarding resident programs and documentation of residents. However, residents may be involved in activities throughout the facility thereby making contact with other activity staff as well. It therefore becomes necessary for the activity staff to share information to help provide up-to-date data on client progress.

Further, several disciplines are commonly involved in providing services to the same clients. Interdisciplinary team meetings also require proper documentation by activity personnel.

Quality Assurance

Quality assurance is a program designed to integrate existing mechanisms of the long-term care facility into a coordinated plan which assures high quality resident care. The quality of care is measured against standards set to achieve optimal results.

Input from sources such as the residents, their family, regulatory agencies and other committees and departments provide data and information which the quality assurance committee identify and study. The results of information received is often based on accurate documentation of problems.

The activity staff plays an important role in documenting resident's progress including goals and plans of residents. Activity personnel are often called upon to respond to family members regarding their relative's participation in therapeutic recreation services. Accurate documentation will provide the quality assurance committee proper information necessary for achieving the best possible resident care.

PAPER WORK REQUIREMENTS

The responsibility for a high level of quality paper work consists of more than the resident care plans and progress notes required by the facility

Table 10-1: Paper Work Requirements

Area of Paper Work	Activity Person Responsible	Required Time for Completion
RECREATION PREFERENCE QUESTIONNAIRE Background assessment Former interests Resident behavior observed Task analysis Family input Resident/family/TRS sign	Activity Leader	Within 10 to 14 days of admission.
VOTER REGISTRATION Resident registers with board of elections for eligibility to vote.	Activity Leader	During interview process.
RESIDENT PHOTOGRAPH To be attached to resident chart in activity file.	Activity Leader	During interview process.
ACTIVITY PARTICIPATION APPROVAL Doctor must approve in writing the level of participation for resident activities.	Activity Leader obtains information previous to interview.	Upon admission.
INITIAL CARE PLAN Problem areas identified. Goals established. Plans developed. Care plan written.	Activity Leader	Following initial interview process.
INDIVIDUALIZED PROGRAM SCHEDULE Specify time/place of desired activities.	Activity Leader	During initial interview.
30-DAY RE-EVALUATION	Activity Leader	Thirty days after admission.
QUARTERLY REVIEW: RESIDENT CARE PLAN/ PROGRESS NOTE Care plan/progress note written. Evaluate goals/assess plans.	Activity Leader	Every three months.
RESIDENT CARE PLAN: Reclassifications	Activity Leader	Upon change or re-classification of resident from one level of care to another.
Return from hospital	Activity Leader	Upon return from hospital.
TEAM MEETING NOTES Team goals/plans	Activity Leader	Yearly.
ATTENDANCE RECORDS/ STATISTICS	Activity Leader Activity Director	Daily/Weekly/Monthly.

Table 10-1: Continued

Area of Paper Work	Activity Person Responsible	Required Time for Completion
PROGRESS REPORT TO ADMINISTRATOR Activities available Resident response to activities. Up-coming plans	Director	Monthly.
DIETARY REQUEST ORDERS	Director	Monthly.
HOUSEKEEPING SET-UP SCHEDULE	Director	Monthly.

and or regulatory agency. In addition, paper work exists at every level of the activity department including the recreation leader and the director. The above table exhibits an overview of the required paper work for most long-term care facilities and delineates responsibility and time elements required for each area. These areas may of course vary, depending upon the type of long-term care facility, its staff complement and the agencies regulating it. A detailed description of paper work requirements and the system utilized for each of these areas will follow.

The Initial Treatment Plan

Recreation preference questionnaire. Upon admission to the long-term care facility every resident needs to be evaluated. This evaluation, which is a mutual process between therapist and resident, helps identify needs, limitations and interests.

The Recreation Preference Questionnaire (see Appendix V) is an evaluative tool used to help identify these needs and interests. Assessing the residents' former interests and involvement in recreational activities, will help provide an overview and a better understanding of the patient's prior lifestyle. This form should be used with the knowledge of the resident's psycho-social profile and medical history usually provided by the social service and nursing departments.

The first meeting between resident and therapist is essential toward establishing an appropriate and successful relationship. Further, it should help provide a supportive atmosphere, conducive to involvement in activities and the entire community of the home or facility.

The meeting needs to be conducted in an atmosphere which promotes conversation and communication and helps to put the resident at ease. Clarity is essential and reassurance is necessary. A genuine concern must be exhibited to help lay the foundation for another support system of the resident.

The recreation leader should use this evaluation as an opportunity to observe the resident's behavior. Resident responses offer significant clues to behaviors and willingness and ability to participate in activities. The therapist must be able to evaluate observations made of the resident which will help identify possible problems related to activity participation.

Task analysis.   Task analysis must also be evaluated during the initial interview. A review of the residents medical history including physical and psychological limitations provides essential information to the therapist. Further, residents may be asked to participate in a certain task which may be necessary for successful participation in an activity. Since this is often a time-consuming process, residents may also be evaluated for participation in specific activities when they attend each activity for the first time.

Family Input.   Since the initial interview is a crucial step toward the foundation of a well developed treatment plan, as much information as possible should be obtained.

It is often helpful to encourage family involvement during the initial interview. Some residents have difficulty in communicating. Some have forgotten past interests or activities they may have enjoyed. Family members may help to fill in the gaps with information useful to the recreation leader. If a family member is unavailable at interview time, a letter to them may indicate interest in their input. At The Jewish Home and Hospital for Aged, a simple, colorful form is given to every family of newly admitted residents with the name and telephone number of the activity director requesting that an appointment be arranged.

Although family members can be helpful a word of caution is advised. Some tend to speak *for* their relative. It may be necessary to encourage the resident to express himself even if his needs do not seem to satisfy his relatives.

Following the interview process, the questionnaire should be signed by the resident (when appropriate), the activity leader and the family member when available.

In summary, the Recreation Preference Questionnaire is a tool utilized to help begin the evaluation process which facilitiates the entire initial treatment/care plan. The questionnaire should therefore include:

Resident background information

Health status

Former interests

Hobbies

Involvement in outside organizations

Available activities at the facility

Available committees or jobs

Voter Registration

The new admission process should include automatic voter registration for residents. Admission to the long-term care facility represents many losses, including work roles, social relationships and material possessions. One social responsibility, the right to vote, need not be lost. It is crucial, therefore, to help the resident carry out this right and obligation.

This is easily achieved if residents are automatically registered upon admission to the facility. Voter registration forms are easily obtained from the local board of elections in most cities.

The activity leader should help the resident complete the registration form which can be sent directly to the Board of Elections. A voter registration book should be kept in the activity department with the name of each resident, who is registered upon admission. This will provide an accurate record of those registered and will alleviate confusion and the need for mass registration previous to annual elections.

Resident Photograph

A photograph of every new resident should be taken and placed into the resident folder kept on file in the activity department. Photographs help identify residents to activity workers and volunteers. They are especially useful in large facilities, helping to identify residents for documentation of resident care plans and progress notes.

Activity Participation Approval

Every resident requires approval from his physician for participation in activities. The level of participation approved by the doctor is an important factor which will influence participation and help determine the treatment care plan. This information should be made available to the activity leader prior to the initial interview process. In addition, every resident should be reviewed by the physician regularly depending upon the requirements of the state code or regulatory agencies affecting the long-term care facility.

Initial Assessment/Care Plan

Following completion of the questionnaire, voter registration, the resident photograph, and activity participation approval, the initial treatment plan is established with the resident and therapist. Included in the treatment plan are specific goals.

The goals are based upon the information received during the interview process utilizing the questionnaire, task analysis, family input and the activity participation approval. Goals should be long and short term as well as realistic and achievable. Goals may also be changeable. Due to their importance, they will be discussed in detail later on in the chapter.

Following the establishment of goals in *writing,* a plan must be developed. The treatment plan will describe *how* goals are to be achieved and will present an overall view of the newly admitted resident.

The following is a typical Initial Assessment Care plan:

> Mrs. R. is an eighty-four-year-old woman who was admitted to the skilled nursing unit due to her need for twenty-four-hour nursing care. She suffers from the beginnings of Alzheimer's disease and although she has some lapse in memory, she remains alert and oriented at this time. Mrs. R. has a history of TIAs, seizures, osteoarthritis and Parkinsonism.
>
> Mrs. R. is a very neat and attractive looking woman who explained during the interview that she did volunteer work and performed professionally as a singer and musician in her former life.
>
> Poor ambulation requires use of a wheelchair. During the interview, Mrs. R. expressed an interest in joining the choral group and musical programs. There seems to be some family involvement and support.
>
> GOAL: To facilitate adjustment to the skilled nursing floor.
>   To establish peer group relationships.
>   To involve Mrs. R. in activities of a musical nature.
>
> PLAN: To invite Mrs. R. to activities, providing her with a weekly activity schedule.
>   To provide escort service to music programs.
>   To seat Mrs. R. near active and sociable residents during activities.

Individualized Activity Schedule

Adjustment to institutionalization is dependent upon a variety of factors. One significant factor is the ability to integrate the resident into the community life of the facility. Thus, participating in activities which provide satisfying experiences are important. A significant part of the initial treatment plan is encouragement of activities the resident expresses an interest in and demonstrates a capability for.

New residents are bombarded with information regarding their environment. Although it is necessary to review the availability of all activities, the new resident needs to be reminded of the time and place of activities he specifically wishes to attend. The individualized activity schedule (see Appendix VI) delineates the time and place of *only those activities the resident wishes to attend.* A copy of this schedule is given to the resident and one is posted on his bulletin board.

Resident Folder

A folder should be maintained in the activities department for each resident. The folder should include copies of pertinent information also filed in the medical chart of each resident. This includes:

Resident photograph
Initial/Assessment care plan
Recreation questionnaire
Nursing and medical history
Social service phycho-social profile
Quarterly resident care plan and progress note
Attendance records if appropriate
Team meeting notes when appropriate

To summarize, the initial assessment and treatment plan procedure should comprise:

Assessment of:

Medical history: past and present
Psycho-social profile

Recreation Preference Questionnaire:

Resident background information
Past interests, past involvement in political organizations or community organizations
Present interests
Available activities and committees at facility
Task analysis

Initial written assessment care plan including:

Specific written goals which identify problem areas and physical and psychological limitations
Specific written plans, describing how goals will be achieved

Activity Participation Approval:

Physician must approve in writing the level of activity participation resident may be involved in.

Figure 10-1 Treatment Plan/Documentation Process

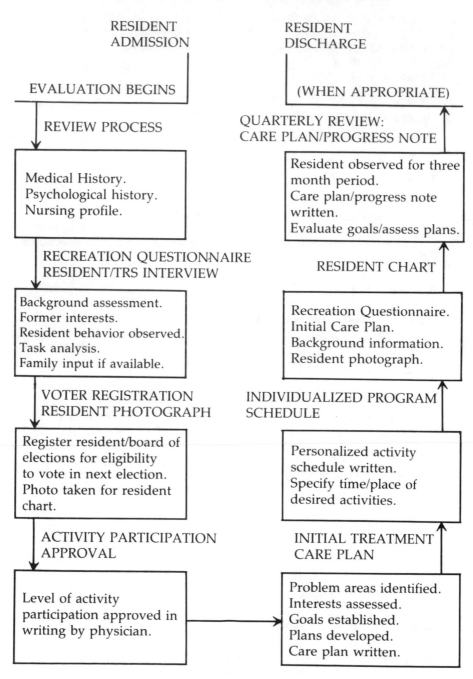

RESIDENT
ADMISSION

EVALUATION BEGINS

REVIEW PROCESS

Medical History.
Psychological history.
Nursing profile.

RECREATION QUESTIONNAIRE
RESIDENT/TRS INTERVIEW

Background assessment.
Former interests.
Resident behavior observed.
Task analysis.
Family input if available.

VOTER REGISTRATION
RESIDENT PHOTOGRAPH

Register resident/board of
elections for eligibility
to vote in next election.
Photo taken for resident
chart.

ACTIVITY PARTICIPATION
APPROVAL

Level of activity
participation approved in
writing by physician.

RESIDENT
DISCHARGE

(WHEN APPROPRIATE)

QUARTERLY REVIEW:
CARE PLAN/PROGRESS NOTE

Resident observed for three
month period.
Care plan/progress note
written.
Evaluate goals/assess plans.

RESIDENT CHART

Recreation Questionnaire.
Initial Care Plan.
Background information.
Resident photograph.

INDIVIDUALIZED PROGRAM
SCHEDULE

Personalized activity
schedule written.
Specify time/place of
desired activities.

INITIAL TREATMENT
CARE PLAN

Problem areas identified.
Interests assessed.
Goals established.
Plans developed.
Care plan written.

Completion of:

Voter registration.
Signing of recreation preference questionnaire
Resident photograph
Completion of resident folder

Following the completion and implementation of the initial assessment treatment/care plan procedure, the resident should be observed for a three month period when his care plan and progress note will be reviewed by the assigned activity leader.

The foregoing illustration denotes the Initial Treatment Plan/Documentation Process.

PATIENT DOCUMENTATION

Common Charting Methods

Format for individual client documentation varies within each facility. Two major procedures are available: the source oriented system and the problem oriented system.[2]

The source oriented system allows for documentation by each individual discipline. Each discipline will have its own section clearly labeled in the resident's medical chart. This system enables each discipline (medical, nursing, occupational therapy, recreation, physical therapy, dietary, etc.) to provide all client documentation in one area. Within the section delineated for each discipline, entries are made which may concern all areas of the client. A progress note may therefore identify several problems related to observations regarding the resident's progress. Although many facilities use this approach, those who oppose the source oriented system believe it takes too long to identify problems since the notes for each discipline must be read separately.

The second system is the problem oriented system. With this system, the medical chart, is organized according to the resident's problem, eliminating separate areas of documentation by each discipline. Those who use the problem oriented approach believe it fosters a greater unification toward individual documentation.

The Resident Care Plan and Progress Note

Regardless of the method used for client documentation, every resident needs to be reviewed periodically and evaluated to examine whether stated goals are being achieved and plans are carried out.

The regulatory bodies governing each agency will usually determine how often residents must be reevaluated.

In New York State, the hospital code requires a specific time frame for reevaluation of residents in activity programs of long-term care facilities. All residents of nursing homes must be reevaluated at least quarterly and the goals and plans must be reviewed as necessary.

Essential Components of Resident Care Plans and Progress Notes

The quarterly review or resident care plan and progress note plays a significant role in the total care of the treatment plan. A review of the essential components of progress notes is warranted.

The progress note indicates information about the resident regarding his progression, regression or apparent change of status, if any is evident. A progress note should contain:

> Information related by the client including any statements he may make regarding problems or feelings he has.
>
> Observations relating problems or facts stated in specific behavioral terms.
>
> i.e.   Resident cried during conversation with recreation leader. She refused to leave the room to attend floor activities.
>
> Positive aspects of resident behavior when they are contributing factors to activity participation.

In addition, the following *specific areas* should also be incorporated into the progress note *when appropriate*. It is important to emphasize that it is not necessary to include every area of concern if it does not relate to the resident or affect his participation in activities.

1.   Medical status:

   Any medical problem or physical limitation related to activity participation or the ability to function should be clearly stated.

   i.e.   CVA, poor vision, hearing impairment.

2.   Psychological status or social behavior:
   i.e.   withdrawn, isolated, sad, happy.

3.   Response to Program:
   i.e.   loner, attends often

4.   Level of participation in the program:
   i.e.   demonstrates leadership abilities, demands attention, active participant.

5. Social interaction and relationships:
    i.e.   socializes with peer group.

6. Attitude:
    i.e.   pleasant, hostile

7. Appearance:
    i.e.   neglects self, clean, neat.

8. Intellectual behavior:
    i.e.   alert, confused, responsive.

9. Team problems and supports:
    i.e.   problems identified by the professional team also need
           to be addressed when appropriate.

All of the above identify certain problem areas and behaviors which determine the level of activity participation, adjustment to the facility and the development of one's leisure lifestyle. Familiarity with these areas is essential in writing effective resident care plans and progress notes. Reference to the above areas will indicate the progress or regression of each resident in achieving his stated goal.

A word of caution is required here. The therapeutic recreation specialist is not qualified to diagnose a specific medical or psychological problem. However, we can identify these problems with a written description of the behaviors which are common to the pathology or illness. For example, we cannot state that a resident is depressed. However, we can state that the resident expresses sadness and cries often.

The following participant behavior index will provide the activity leader with a variety of phrases to be utilized in writing effective care plans and progress notes.

Goals and Plans

Goals and plans are an essential component of the resident care plan and progress note. All identified problems require intervention and treatment which result in the setting of goals. The following guidelines will be helpful in setting goals. Goals should be:

1. Individualized and should relate to the particular area
    identified for intervention or treatment.
    i.e.   an identified problem may be that a resident participates in a music program but will not hold a musical
           instrument.
    GOAL: Get resident to hold tambourine during music
           program for five minutes.

Table 10-2: Participant Behavior Index

Participation:
arrives late
socializes but does not participate in
    activity
socializes with peers
active participant
passive participant
enjoys activity
dislikes activity
attends regularly
attends occasionally

Social Behavior:
avoids opposite sex
member of "clique"
self-conscious
outgoing and friendly
impolite
withdrawn
unpopular with others
acts out
likeable
fearful and uncertain
monopolizes one's attention

Performance:
capable of doing well if interested
perfectionist
eager to learn
not very skilled
performs well

Appearance:
neat and well-groomed
looks tired
sloppy, unkempt
inappropriately dressed
appropriately dressed

Attitudes:
anxious
hostile
cooperative
withdrawn
manipulative

Physical Behavior:
smokes, drinks
relaxes
reserved
restless
overactive

Mood:
good-natured disposition
bored
angry
elated
upsets easily
appears sad
has mood changes
tearful
preoccupied

Intellectual Behavior:
appears self-confident
forgetful
doesn't pay attention
alert and responsive
confused
demonstrates poor judgement

Communication:
talks to staff only
talks only to participants
uses strange words
overtalkative
hesitant, uncertain in speech
responsive on approach
unresponsive
logical, coherent
sarcastic
vulgar

Miscellaneous:
neglects responsibilities
has many physical complaints
hard to please
well adjusted
suspicious

2. Achieveable and realistic:

    Unrealistic goals will result in frustration for both the participant and the activity leader.

    For the above goal to be achieved, the resident must be able to hold the instrument. In addition, the time limit (five minutes) must be realistically set based upon the attention span and mental ability of the resident.

3. Measurable:

    The goal must be measureable.
    i.e. we must be able to observe and measure whether the
          resident in fact was able to hold the instrument for
          five minutes.

4. Specific:

    Goals must be specific. The above goals identifies a specific
    action or behavior which needs to be accomplished.

Many facilities require long and short term goals. Whether or not they are
required, it is helpful to think of goals as short or long term.

    i.e. long-term goal: increase socialization.
          short-term goal: get resident to respond during one
                            to one contact.

    Plans must be written for every progress note and these usually follow
the written goals. The plan describes *how* you wish to achieve your stated
goals. The type of intervention and the techniques used will be described
in the plan. A plan should be:

1. Related to the stated goal.
    i.e. Goal: Get resident to hold and shake the tambourine
                 for five minutes.
         Plan: Instruct resident on how to hold and shake the
                 tambourine during the program. Sit resident next
                 to someone who can assist her with the instru-
                 ment.

    This plan relates to its goal by describing techniques which
    will help achieve the stated goal.

2. Realistic and achievable:

    This plan is both realistic and achieveable in that the res-
    ident is being offered instruction and is not expected to
    learn how to use this instrument on her own.

3. Specific:

    The plan should state specific procedures to help accom-
    plish its goal.

    Goals and Plans are often confused. The following will help to distin-
guish between goals and plans.

A *goal* describes: *what* specific objective you wish to accomplish.

A *plan* describes: *how* you will accomplish your goal.

The following list provides long and short term goals which can be utilized by the activity leader in the documentation of resident care plans and progress notes.

Goals:

Promote perceptual-motor coordination.

Achieve proper use of leisure time.

Increase sensory awareness.

Increase attention span.

Increase auditory awareness.

Decrease social isolation.

Increase opportunity for social contact.

Provide opportunity for non-verbal communication.

Increase non-verbal communication responses.

Increase communication skills.

Stimulate cognitive functioning.

Stimulate physical abilities.

Establish positive relationship with activity worker.

Resident will give eye contact.

Resident will throw ball.

Resident will hold rhythm instrument.

It should be noted that effective documentation includes resident care plans for clients whose status or classification changes. Any resident who is re-classified to a higher or lower level of care requires a new evaluation and treatment care plan. Residents who return from outside hospitals also require a review of their treatment plan.

To summarize, the essential ingredients of the Resident Care Plan are the statements regarding the progression toward or regression from goal achievement. Comprising these statements are factors relating to the residents' medical status and physical and/or psychological limitations. Consideration also needs to be given to:

Response to the program.

Level of participation in program.

Social interaction and relationship with peer and staff.

Attitude.

Behavior patterns.

Team supports.

The combination of these ingredients as well as certain outside factors seem to influence the focus or emphasis of the resident care plan. Such factors include standards set by the long-term care facility often mandated by its regulatory agencies.

RESOURCE UTILIZATION GROUPINGS

The recent implementation of a new reimbursement system for long-term care facilities (RUGS) developed in New York State is having great implications for the documentation of treatment plans and progress notes in therapeutic recreation.

A brief overview of the RUGS II system is warranted to help provide the rationale for a change in focus in documentation of resident care plans for therapeutic recreation.

The cost of long-term care has risen dramatically in the last twenty years. Rates in New York State have traditionally been based on the calculation of historical cost which reflects an amount required to run the facility. Increases were based upon the estimated inflation rate with a ceiling set for cost containment. However, the impact of the patient mix was not accounted for in calculating facility costs. Nursing homes received the same reimbursement for all patients regardless of the amount of care they required. As a result, many homes refused patients requiring heavier care.

Thus, the implementation of RUGS II addresses patient mix in the long-term care facility in relation to a more equitable distribution of money. This system will, therefore, allow sicker patients easier access to the long-term care facility. Because of its broad applicability, the system may also be used for quality of care, staffing, utilization review and other related areas.

The RUGS II system was funded by a grant from the United States department of Health and Human Services (DHHS) and the Health Care Financing Administration. (HCFA) New York State provided additional funds. The system was developed as part of the long-term care case mix reimbursement project and is being run under the auspices of the New York State department of Health and the School of Management at Rensselear Polytechnic Institute. The concept of case mix reimbursement has been gaining acceptance over the years. Thus, implementation of the system could easily take place in states throughout the nation.

The main goal of the case mix project was to develop a patient classification system that "defines groups of patients according to similar clinical characteristics and resource consumption."[3] Since nursing staff provides the bulk of the "hands on" care, the RUGS system evaluates the amount of nursing care or resources required for the patients clinical condition. The amount of care required is then translated into reimbursement needs.

The RUGS system is the result of data collected from over 3400 residents in fifty-two New York State facilities.[4] The combination of data and clinical input from experts in the long-term care field lead to the RUGS II system. This system is composed of five major clinical groups which are further subdivided, using ADL's (activities of daily living) into sixteen groups. The five clinical groups are:[5]

1. Special Care
2. Rehabilitation
3. Clinical Complex
4. Severe Behavioral Problems
5. Reduced Physical Functioning

In order to translate the amount of care required into the amount of money needed, an assessment of the patient is necessary. The Patient Review Instrument (PRI) obtains information to help place the patient into the appropriate RUGS category. The PRI addresses:

1. Medical events including conditions and treatments.
2. Activities of daily living including: eating, mobility, transfer and toileting.
3. Behaviors (disruptive and nondisruptive) including:

    verbal disruption, physical aggression, infantile or socially inappropriate behavior, hallucinations.
4. Specialized services including:

    physical therapy, occupational therapy.

The resulting data of the PRI forms are reviewed by specially trained case mix nurses who provide on-site reviews at each facility. These reviews confirm the actual condition of the patient within the time period and frequency required by the RUGS system. Interviews with staff, observation of residents and evaluation of documentation are included in the on-site review process.

The importance of documenting the amount of clinical care needed for residents now becomes significant on every level and in every discipline including therapeutic recreation.

For example, the resident who cannot eat without assistance will also presumably require help at a recreation activity such as a barbecue. Although we may have considered assisting residents at barbecues a natural function of our job, the RUGS system facilitates mention of events such as these.

Many residents require staff time and assistance at activities due to verbal and/or physical disruptions. Although we have handled these types of situations before, documentation may have not always reflected these instances.

In addition, we are now asked to log any behavioral or care related problem which requires staff intervention or time with particular residents.

The RUGS II system is changing the *focus* of our resident care plans and documentation requirements. In essence, notes are becoming a support system showing continuity of required care *when and if* it relates to the therapeutic environment and activity program. It is important to remember, however, that *not every resident may have a RUGS issue related to activities*.

It is important for the activity leader to be aware of the system, providing accurate documentation related both to therapeutic recreation needs and RUGS related issues.

TEAM MEETINGS

Interdisciplinary team meetings are also an important part of the residents' treatment plan.

In addition to the individualized resident care plan written by the therapeutic recreation specialist, team goals are essential for the care of the patient.

Every agency differs in its approach to the team meeting and its goals. The activity leader may be asked to participate in identifying resident problems as part of the team or he may be asked to identify problems listing them separately.

Whatever system is used, the activity leader should incorporate team goals into the quarterly resident care plan and progress note when appropriate.

DOCUMENTATION: A SYSTEMATIZED APPROACH

Documentation consists of more than effective note writing. Activity leaders must know when to write notes on their assigned residents. Some activity directors allow their workers to use their own system, seldom reviewing notes except for occasional audits.

Paper work is time consuming and should be viewed as a "process." A systematized approach to care plan distribution, note writing and auditing will provide the most accurate and efficient time system possible.

At The Jewish Home and Hospital for Aged, Bronx, New York, the following method has proved successful for over 820 residents.

A file box is used which holds a 3 x 5 index card with each resident's name, room number and date indicating when each care plan is due. Since each resident must be reviewed every three months (New York State hospital code requirements), the cards are divided by month for a three-month period (i.e. January, February, March). Within each month the cards are subdivided into sections by the number of weeks in each month. In each weekly section, the cards are placed according to *room number* rather than alphabetically. Thus, changes in room numbers by resident transfers and/ or deaths, merely require moving the card to a different part of the same section in the box.

Two separate file boxes with two different colored cards are used; one for Health Related residents and one for Skilled Nursing residents. Thus, changes in classification require a new card to be made and placed in the appropriate box and month which will indicate when the care plan must be written.

A list is written weekly for each activity leader on a specially devised form (See Appendix VII for Resident Care Plan Review and Audit system form) delineating which residents are due for care plans. Space is provided on the list for the activity leader to initial completion of his notes. In addition, a space is provided on the list so that while the activity leader is at each medical chart he can audit and check the team meeting notes, the recreation questionnaire, the last quarterly resident care plan and the physicians approval for activity participation. Upon completion, the list of all care plans for the week is returned to the director. The date of the care plan listed on each file card is now crossed off by the director and put into the month denoting the next three-month period or cycle. It should be noted that the date listed on the file card is always a Monday. This allows the activity leader a week in which to complete his assigned care plans.

The following illustration denotes the Resident Care Plan Distribution and Audit Review System.
This system has several advantages:

1. The director maintains an accurate account of which residents require care plans and progress notes.

2. The activity leader is not left to chance, guessing when notes are due for residents.

3. The audit system built into the specially devised form, ensures that all care plans and other required paper work is completed throughout the year. This facilitates completion of state code requirements examined during the state survey process.

4. Changes in classification of residents are easily handled. New color coded cards are completed for any classification change. This ensures that no residents fall between the cracks.

Figure 10-2 Resident Care Plan Distribution and Audit Review System

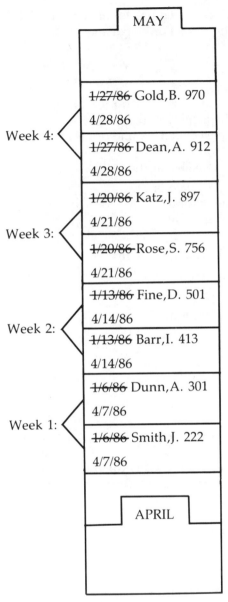

Figure 1:
Resident Care Plan
File Cards

Resident Care Plan
Distribution/Audit System.

Name:	Room:	Date:
Smith, J.	222	4/7/
Dunn, A.	301	4/7/

Figure 2: Resident name
written on weekly list.

Care Plan	Team Meet.	Act. App.	Rec. Quest.	TRS Initial
✓	✓	✓	✓	F. G.

Figure 3: TRS initials completion of care plans in last
column and check appropriate
boxes for auditing.

File Card

~~1/6/86~~	J. Smith	222
~~4/7/86~~		
7/6/87		

Figure 4: Activity director
reviews list and audits.
Completed care plan date
(4/7/86) is crossed off.
Card re-dated for three
months and filed.

ADDITIONAL DOCUMENTATION REQUIREMENTS

In addition to individual client documentation, other types of paper work are required in many therapeutic recreation departments.

Progress Report to Administrator

An efficient director will keep his administrator up to date regarding the progress, changes and plans of the activity department.

The progress report should be completed monthly and usually includes:

1. A list of activities currently available at the facility.
2. A short summary when appropriate on:
    special events of the previous month.
    holiday parties of the previous month.
    outings which took place
3. An outline of plans for the upcoming months.
4. Resident response to the program.
5. A calendar of events for the following month.
6. Any problems you may wish the administrator to be aware of.

The Progress Report should be signed and dated by the activity director.

Policy and Procedure Manual

An updated procedure manual is not only required by the state hospital code, but it provides efficient administrative functioning. The procedure manual, which should be updated yearly, provides for the review and evaluation of policies and procedures of the activity department.

The manual should include:

1. A philosophy of the department.
2. Goals of the department.
3. Resident activity policies.
4. Structure and operation of the department.
5. Activity department forms.
6. Attendance procedures and forms.
7. Voter registration procedures.
8. Activity planning procedures.

9. Administrative practices:
   organizational chart
   budget
   inventory
   housekeeping schedule for setups
   dietary requests
   purchasing procedures
   maintenance and repairs
   state survey procedures
   job descriptions
   religious procedures and practices
10. Staffing patterns.
11. Volunteer services procedures.
    evaluations, recruitment, etc.

Attendance Records and Statistical Reports

Statistical reports of resident participation at activities are usually required by the activities department and or regulatory agencies.

Methods for maintaining attendance records will vary. Attendance records for small group activities (5–25) usually include resident names. Attendance for large group activities (25 or more) usually do not require the names of those who attend.

Accurate attendance records and statistics are necessary for several reasons:

1. Attendance patterns provide significant information for completing care plans and progress notes.
2. Attendance records are partial indicators of the popularity of certain activities.
3. Attendance statistics provide information to administration for rationalization of certain activity programs.
4. Attendance statistics are utilized by the accounting department for reimbursement purposes.
5. Attendance statistics are required by several regulatory agencies.

Staff Meetings and Minutes

Staff meetings are essential in maintaining effective communication among staff.

Meetings should be held on a regular basis and should include:

1. Activity planning sessions
2. Program evaluation
3. Staff evaluations
4. Supervision and training sessions
5. In-service sessions

Accurate minutes should be kept for reference purposes. In addition, many regulatory agencies and state codes require minutes of staff meetings.

STATE SURVEY

Long-term care facilities have long felt the implications and effects of the guidelines and standards set by the local, state and federal governments.

As trends change within the long-term care facilities, so do the processes by which surveys and inspections are conducted. Present changes represent alterations in evaluative procedures which now focus on resident care rather than on paper work policies and procedures. Thus, examining patient care from a variety of perspectives adds new challenges to the delivery of health care within the long-term care facility.

Guidelines and surveys vary from state to state. A new system has been implemented in New York State as of April 1, 1986. PaCS (Patient Care and Services) will evaluate nursing homes and long-term care facilities, examining patient care areas with greater scrutiny than before.

Previous to PaCS, the structural requirements of the nursing home (cleanliness, safety, environmental factors, etc.) were often equated with the quality of care received by the residents. However, several studies began to show that structure and quality were in fact not always equal and therefore could not be equated with better or worse resident care.[6] PaCs was, therefore, developed to provide greater validity and more credibility to the survey process.[7]

Although paper work will still be evaluated, the survey will focus on resident centered care which will include on-site interviews with residents, staff and family members when available. Tours and observations of activities, drug distribution and dietary services will also be implemented.

It is crucial for the activity director to maintain awareness and knowledge of the state code requirements and survey process both presently and as it changes.

PaCs represents a variety of changes and challenges for the activity department.

Although paper work will still be examined, on site observations of activities in progress will also be conducted. Residents will be interviewed to be sure their interests are being met through the availability of a meaningful activities program. In addition to observation of activities in progress, the surveyor will observe resident rooms, noting pictures, crafts projects or other articles which may indicate the level of involvement within activities and the quality of life they are afforded.

Interviews of residents will also be conducted by the surveyors. These will address the following issues:

1. The resident will be given the opportunity of discussing how they spend their time.

2. The resident will be asked if they are aware of available activities and special events.

3. The resident will be asked if transportation to and from activities is available if necessary.

4. The resident will be asked if they are afforded opportunities to relate to the outside community through outings, etc.

Through the PaCS survey there should be evidence that the resident is involved in meaningful activities which satisfy individualized resident needs. Follow up, goals and plans are essential in maintaining progress for all residents.

SUMMARY

Documentation plays a significant role in the delivery of therapeutic recreation services. To dismiss the importance of documentation is to ignore our responsibilities and accountability as professionals. An understanding of documentation skills within a systematized process will help provide the highest possible level of therapeutic recreation services.

Justification for documentation and a belief in its importance is essential to the activity director.

A concise understanding of required paper work such as the recreation questionnaire, the initial treatment care plan, the quarterly review, progress reports and attendance statistics is necessary.

Familiarity with the state code and regulatory bodies governing the agency is equally important. The implications for the activities department of such codes and regulatory standards must be clearly understood.

Finally, a systematized process for documentation requirements will provide maximum effectiveness for both the department and its staff.

FILLING THE GLASS WITH POTENTIAL

The process of aging is inevitable. How we age is not.

Aging is concomitant with change. Biological aging results in changes such as wrinkles, the loss of teeth and the graying of hair. Disease processess may result in further changes such as deformities due to arthritis or osteoporosis.

A second type of aging also exists: aging due to "stereotypes" and "roles." This type of aging seems to produce changes as well. These changes, however, represent attitudes which are manifested in the negative roles assigned to the aged based upon chronological age.

Mandatory retirement seems to be synonymous with the inability of maintaining one's "normal" functioning level merely because one has "come of age." Our youth oriented culture has created a society afraid of growing old. The elderly are supposed to become ill, unproductive and useless once they reach retirement age. They are seen as lonely and weak, slow to learn and not very intelligent. In fact, the aged are often pitied.

So deep rooted are these negative stereotypes, that even the "old" people of our society believe in them. It is no wonder that admission to the long-term care facility or nursing home represents to many a "resting place" for the elderly whose roles have already been defined for them by society. "I'm too old and too sick to do anything" is a cry often heard in the nursing home.

The views of aging in America and their negative stereotypes remain as obstacles to the goals and philosophy of therapeutic recreation services. The delivery of therapeutic recreation services depends upon the development of leisure skills and attitudes toward leisure involvement. A more positive image of and by the aged, would help change attitudes necessary to the development of an appropriate leisure lifestyle. As Alex Comfort indicates:

> The changes which could remedy this deficit and evoke the full intellectual and physical powers which human beings possess lifelong, are changes of attitudes. Once an older person comes to be seen, not as old first and provisionally a person second, but as a person who happens also to be old, and who is still as he or she always was, plus experience and minus the consequences of certain physical accidents of time, only then will social gerontology have made its point.[1]

It is essential to help the aged person facilitate changes in attitudes which will allow him to utilize the services of therapeutic recreation to a greater extent.

The aged need to see themselves in a more positive light. How many view the half filled glass as half empty? We need to look at the glass as an opportunity of filling it with the resources and potentials of aging and life.

We need to view the glass as the chance to further our growth, accept change and offer positive responses to the obstacles of aging. No one can deny the biological changes and physical problems which become increasingly prevalent with age. Problems won't just disappear. However, a positive outlook and optimum leisure involvement will help to lessen the *preoccupation* with the *symptoms* of old age.

Helping the elderly to use the strengths of life's resources will help to fill the glass with potential. New strengths can be used to build new skills. The elderly need to accept responsibility in how they age. Their attitudes and outlook, as well as that of society's, will influence the positive effects provided through the delivery of therapeutic recreation services.

APPENDICES

PHILOSOPHICAL POSITION STATEMENT
National Therapeutic Recreation Society

Leisure, including recreation and play, is an inherent aspect of the human experience. The importance of appropriate leisure involvement has been documented throughout history. More recently, research has addressed the value of leisure involvement in human development, in social and family relationships, and, in general, as an important aspect of the quality of life. Some human beings have disabilities, illnesses or social conditions which limit their full participation in the normative social structure of society. These individuals with limitations have the same human rights to, and needs for, leisure involvement.

The purpose of therapeutic recreation is to facilitate the development, maintenance, and expression of an appropriate leisure lifestyle for individuals with physical, mental, emotional or social limitations. Accordingly, this purpose is accomplished through the provision of professional programs and services which assist the client in eliminating barriers to leisure, developing leisure skills and attitudes and optimizing leisure involvement. Therapeutic recreation professionals use these principles to enhance clients' leisure ability in recognition of the importance and value of leisure in the human experience.

Three specific areas of professional services are employed to provide this comprehensive leisure ability approach toward enabling appropriate leisure lifestyles: therapy, leisure education, and recreation participation. While these three areas of service have unique purposes in relation to client need, they each employ similar delivery processes, using assessment or identification of client need, development of a related program strategy, and monitoring and evaluating client outcomes. The decision regarding where and when each of the three service areas would be provided is based on the assessment of client needs and the service mandate of the sponsoring agency. The selection of appropriate service areas is contingent on a recognition that different clients have differing needs related to leisure involvement in view of their personal life situation.

The purpose of the therapy service area within therapeutic recreation is to improve functional behaviors. Some clients may require treatment or remediation of afunctional behavior as a necessary prerequisite to enable their involvement in meaningful leisure experiences. Therapy, therefore, is viewed as most appropriate when clients have functional limitations that relate to, or inhibit, their potential leisure involvement. This distinction enables the therapeutic recreator to decide when therapy service is appropriate, as well as to identify the types of behaviors that are most appropriate to address within the therapeutic recreation domain of expertise and authority. In settings where a comprehensive treatment approach is used, therapy focuses on team-identified treatment goals, as well as addressing unique aspects of leisure-related functional behaviors. This approach places therapeutic recreation as an integral and cooperative member of the comprehensive treatment team, while linking its primary focus to eventual leisure ability.

The purpose of the leisure education service is to provide opportunities for the acquisition of skills, knowledge and attitudes related to leisure involvement. For some clients, acquiring leisure skills, knowledge and attitudes are priority needs. It appears that the majority of clients in residential, treatment and community settings need leisure education services in order to initiate and engage in leisure experiences. It is the absence of leisure learning opportunities and socialization into leisure that blocks or inhibits these individuals from participation in leisure experiences. Here, leisure education services would be employed to provide the client with leisure skills, to enhance the client's attitudes concerning the value and importance of leisure, as well as learning about opportunities and resources for leisure involvement. Thus, leisure education programs provide the opportunity for the development of leisure behaviors and skills.

The purpose of the recreation participation area of therapeutic recreation services is to provide opportunities which allow voluntary client involvement in recreation interests and activities. Human beings, despite disability, illness or other limiting conditions, and regardless of place of residence, are entitled to recreation opportunities. The justification for specialized recreation participation programs is based on the clients' need for assistance and or adapted recreation equipment, limitations imposed by restrictive treatment or residential environments, or the absence of appropriate community recreation opportunities. In therapeutic recreation services, the need for recreation participation is acknowledged and given appropriate emphasis in recognition of the intent of the leisure ability concept.

These three service areas of therapeutic recreation represent a continuum of care, including therapy, leisure education and the provision of special recreation participation opportunities. This comprehensive leisure ability approach uses the need of the client to give direction to program service selection. In some situations, the client may need programs for all three service areas. In other situations, the patient may require only one or two of the service areas.

Equally important is the concern of generalizing therapeutic recreation services across the diverse service delivery settings. The leisure ability approach of therapeutic recreation provides appropriate program direction regardless of type of setting or type of client served. A professional working in a treatment setting can see the extension of the leisure ability approach toward client needs within the community environment. Likewise, those within the community can view therapeutic recreation services within a perspective of previous services received or possible future needs.

All human beings, including those individuals with disabilities, illnesses or limiting conditions, have a right to, and a need for, leisure involvement as a necessary aspect of the human experience. The purpose of therapeutic recreation services is to facilitate the development, maintenance, and expression of an appropriate leisure lifestyle for individuals with limitations through the provision of therapy, leisure education, and recreation participation services. The National Therapeutic Recreation Society is the acknowledged professional organization representing the field of therapeutic recreation. The NTRS exists to foster the development and advancement of this field in order to ensure quality professional services and to protect the rights of consumers of therapeutic recreation services. In order to provide consistent and identifiable services throughout the field, the National Therapeutic Recreation Society endorses the leisure ability philosophy described herein as the official position statement regarding therapeutic recreation.

THE PERSONALIZED CARE MODEL FOR THE ELDERLY

The Personalized Care Model (PCM) is a multidimensional system that integrates resources of the facility to achieve delivery of quality and humanistic care to the institutionalized elderly. It insures that the care plan is holistically conceptualized and that services and programming are personalized. The system brings to patient and staff alike a sense of dignity often lacking in traditional models that tend to address a single diagnosis or disability rather than the whole person in his environment. The theories and perspectives underlying the development of PCM stem from the works of the cultural anthropologists.

PCM CONSISTS OF:

a methodology of staff education and organization;

a methodology of unit management;

a methodology of environmental management;

a methodology and techniques for individualizing patient care and achieving quality assurance;

a philosophy and methodology for patient activities, program design, and program management;

techniques and guidelines for implementation of the system.

FOUNDATIONS OF THE PERSONALIZED CARE MODEL

The initial work that led to the development of the Personalized Care Model was made possible by a grant from the National Institute of Mental Health (NIMH).[1] In accordance with the guidelines specified on the request for proposal, a two part project was proposed by the Department of Anthropology of Syracuse University's Utica College;[2] namely, the development of a multidisciplinary curriculum, and the training of all levels of staff of long term-care facilities in the Utica, New York area. Participants were to be drawn from skilled nursing and health-related facilities, adult homes, and geriatric wards of a state psychiatric center and an acute-care facility. As part of the process of determining the educational needs of these potential participants, four anthropologists were assigned to a number of the facilities expressing interest in the project to identify both real and perceived educational needs. Data were collected by means of surveys and participant observation.

In the course of this study, in addition to identifying training needs, certain aspects of the culture and environment were recorded, aspects that appeared to strongly influence patient outcome and behavior in the institution. At the end of the first year, when it was found that education of staff was not appreciably changing staff performance or patient behavior, the anthropologists returned to these facilities to study the situation further and to identify barriers to change.

Findings from this second wave of contacts made it evident that the culture was derived primarily from the medical model of care, interaction and delivery of services. Staff were educated and trained according to the patterns of this model to attend to certain *tasks,* disabilities, or problems, not the whole person. Focus of care was on the body and the preservation of the body's life. A minimal amount of attention was directed to the mind and meaningful activities of the mind.

Data indicated also that the myths and misconceptions about aging and the aged as well as many gaps in knowledge of the respective disciplines mitigated against providing meaningful programming or activities for the institutionalized. This situation was exacerbated by a number of state policies that were aimed at protecting the patient; the by-product, however, was marked role diminishment for the patient.

Staff organization and interpersonal relationships were such that they reinforced and perpetuated the medical aspects of the culture while limiting the focus on all other aspects of the person. This focus was seen as destructive to the individual at both the biological-physiological and the psychological-social levels. For instance, the dependency relationship between staff and patients often precluded the initiation of bodily activities at a higher level, or the maintenance of such activities at a pre-institutional level. Deculturation and role diminshement were seen as significant factors in the onset of withdrawal, confusion, and memory loss.

The physical environment was perceived by staff only minimally as a factor that contributed to the patients' physical and mental well-being. It was not clearly recognized as a potential source of problems or as a resource for solutions of problems. For instance, isolation and withdrawal of patients were not addressed by such actions as clustering of chairs or moving them away from walls in corridors. Lighting and glare were seldom considered as causes of hallucinatory behaviors. High levels of noise were not recognized as causative of such behaviors as agitation and wandering.

Meaningful activities for patients were limited and this role diminishement led to withdrawal and cognitive decline that was not caused by biological and physiological deterioration. Activities tended to be large scale and separating (bingo, sing-a-longs), standardized and gereralized, off the floors, particularized to "good" patients, available at particular times (staff preference), and determined by staff. A limited number of patients were seen to participate in available activities. Others were involved in no activities save nursing-station watching.

The totality of findings indicated that if significant changes in staff performance or patient behavior were to be achieved, changes in the traditional system must be accomplished. Interventions must be initiated in those areas that impacted so critically on patient outcome in the institution; namely, the knowledge base, physical environment, interpersonal relationships, social interaction and involvement in meaningful activities, and staff organization. In response to this hypothesis, intervention objectives were delineated and strategies to bring about change were conceptualized. Over the subsequent years of NIMH funding, these strategies were field tested (1977–1981). In this manner, from the initial educational project, over time, the Personalized Care Model evolved.

SYSTEMS CHANGE

Implementation of the Personalized Care Model requires changes in five areas of the institution:

1.   the cultural milieu
2.   the physical environment

3. the social structure
4. the nature of activities or programming
5. the organizational structure

I. CULTURAL CHANGE: OBJECTIVES OF INTERVENTION

1. to present a multidisciplinary training that provides staff with a current knowledge base concerning the aged and the aging process, and a holistic perspective of the elder as a unique human being;
2. to present the theoretical foundations of the Personalized Care Model, its philosophy, principles, and objectives;
3. to develop an awareness on the part of staff of the cultural predispositions of the elderly in their facility;
4. to develop a sensitivity to the impact of physical environment on physical and mental well-being of the institutionalized;
5. to develop an awareness of, and sensitivity to, nonverbal communication, its impact upon resident behavior and orientation, and its significance with respect to understanding that behavior;
6. to modify attitudes and expectations of staff with respect to their roles and patient potential;
7. to develop staff skills in facilitating the role transitions that are part of the institutionalization process.

II. PHYSICAL ENVIRONMENTAL CHANGE: OBJECTIVES OF INTERVENTION

1. to increase staff awareness of the physical environment as an integral part of the humanizing services;
2. to increase staff awareness of the physical environment as a potential source of wide-ranging problems and as a resource for creating a more supportive environment;
3. to make available a variety of settings that stimlate mental activity, facilitate social interaction, and make possible bodily activities, motion, and exercise;
4. to modify the physical environment to provide multidimensional supports to sensory or cognitively impaired patients.
5. to provide spaitial options for patients, staff and families with respect to size of social group gatherings;
6. to make available space, materials, and furniture that is supportive of the respective needs of patients.

III. SOCIAL CHANGE: OBJECTIVES OF INTERVENTION

1. to individualize and personalize patient care by restructuring the patterns of inter-personal relationships;
2. to set up patterns of interaction that ensure continuity and accountability;

3. to modify the roles of direct care givers and reorder patterns of reciprocity;

4. to reorder traditional aide-patient relationships to achieve PCM relationships, i.e:

Traditional	*PCM*
dependency	helping
task-oriented	person-oriented
problem-oriented	potential-oriented
custodial care	meaningful activities
discontinuity	bridging
diffuse assignments	stabilized
non-accountability	assignment
fragmentation	accountability
	continuity

5. to reorder professional paraprofessional roles and relationships.

IV.   PROGRAMMING CHANGE: OBJECTIVES OF INTERVENTION

1. to diminish or prevent spatial isolation and/or withdrawal of patients;

2. to involve patients, to the fullest extent possible, in adaptive activities, social interaction, and personally meaningful experiences;

3. to make available standard activities/programs to all patients, in accord with level of functioning and in a variety of settings;

4. to develop meaningful activities that are personalized to patient interests and level of functioning;

5. to establish activity groups for small numbers of patients in accordance with their interests, capabilities, and life-long inclinations;

6. to utilize staff and patients to provide leadership for small group-interest activities.

V.   ORGANIZATIONAL CHANGE: OBJECTIVES OF INTERVENTION

1. to establish an administrative and functional structure in the institution to operationalize the Personalized Care Model system;

2. to designate staff for PCM positions and establish lines of reporting, namely, the Primary Helper role (aide), the PCM Implementor (administrative) and PCM Facilitators (clinical);

3. to operationalize behavior associated with PCM positions;

4. to establish reciprocity between traditional and PCM positions and roles;

5. to establish a system whereby the primary helper is stablized to a cluster of patients and represents those cluster members in multidisciplinary team meetings;

6. to establish a multidiciplinary (departmental) implementing committee and functional subcommittees.

PCM Field Testing

Connecticut

The first broad testing of PCM occurred in Connecticut[3] (1978–1981) where the project was housed for two years at the University of Connecticut and a final year with the State Department of Mental Health. A number of strategies for accomplishing state-wide replications were developed and tested. PCM was implemented in a number of long-term care facilities and was designated as the method of care delivery for geriatric patients in two of the state hospitals.

When federal funding ceased, Norwich Hospital took on the responsibility for PCM dissemination. Since 1981, staff at the hospital have continued to mount training-implementation workshops and to provide clinical experiences for trainees throughout the state.

New York State Office of Mental Health

In 1981, PCM staff returned to New York State where the system was sponsored by the Office of Mental Health (OMH). Designated as the approach to be used on geriatric wards,[4] the system was introduced (1981–1983) across the state and was implemented in eleven psychiatric centers. OMH's policy of outreach made it possible for the staff of long-term care facilities to participate in workshops mounted in the state facilities.

By 1984, under a mandate from the Long Island Regional Director,[5] training and implementation of PCM was begun at all four of the region's facilities and for all populations. Modification of the curriculum was undertaken for the younger adult and the children and youth populations by clinicians working with the respective populations and the Director of the Personalized Care Model.[6] Comprehensive evaluation of this new application of PCM is being accomplished by a team of researchers.

Veterans Hospital

Also, in 1984, with training of key staff accomplished in the area psychiatric center, implementation of PCM was begun on demonstration wards at the Montrose Veterans Hospital, Montrose, New York. Impetus came from the nursing department.[7] In early 1985, a comprehensive training program was initiated at the hospital to prepare other staff in the system. Plans have been introduced to extend the system to other wards and to the psychogeriatric patients.

Nursing Homes

From 1975 to 1985, staff from nursing homes made up approximately one third of the five thousand trainees and a representative number of these participants returned to their respective facilities to implement PCM. It was not, however, until 1983 that a large multi-level nursing home adopted the system. In the fall of that year, The Jewish Home and Hospital for Aged, Kingsbridge Center, in the Bronx,

New York, mounted requisite training and initiated PCM on two demonstration floors in a skilled nursing unit.

In 1984, six additional floors began the initial phase of implementation. By 1985, plans were underway to extend the system to the Manhattan division of The Jewish Home and Hospital for Aged (Central House). Prior to the introduction of the PCM at Central House, however, data is being gathered as the basis for a comprehensive multidimensional evaluation of the process of implementation and its outcome in a nursing home setting. The ultimate objective of the research is to increase knowledge about long-term care practices and methods for promoting mental and physical functioning of elderly nursing home residents.

The research will test several hypotheses with respect to the impact of PCM on a number of aspects of resident functioning and staff behavior. Both quantitative and qualitative methodologies will be employed. It is anticipated that the study will be completed in late 1987 although some preliminary results may be available late in 1986.

PCM Implementation Outcome

Findings from earlier evaluations that were primarily qualitative in nature, have shown that implementation of PCM ensures total accountability on the part of staff, increases staff morale, significantly modifies staff attitudes and expectations and reduces staff turnover and absenteeism.

For a significant number of patients, the Personalized Care Model system alleviates symptoms that replicate senile dementia and significantly reduces confusion, memory loss and withdrawal. Levels of functioning are increased and an environment is created in which staff-patient verbal interaction more nearly approaches a status-equality relationship.[8] Implementation also eliminates many attributes that are part of the "patient-sick" role, decreases dependency in activities of daily living and increases decision making.

Overall, PCM improves the quality of life of the resident and enhances the dignity of both resident and staff.

Additional observations from outside the OMH system come from such sources as the Joint Commission for the Accreditation of Hospitals (JCAH). Surveyors have stated for the record that the PCM "encompasses the essence of the standards with regard to patients' rights, with regard to therapeutic environment and in regard to the morale of staff and the enthusiasm of staff that all have to be present in any treatment facility in order to carry out the program"[9] or again in 1984, ". . . There is an attitude here that is conveyed at every level as PCM is enthusiastically embraced by the staff. The whole place changes . . . and . . . picks up enormously (as staff expectations of patients become positive) compared to the non PCM wards where work with the chronic patient is accomplished without much hope in what is being done.

Modification in behavior of patients on PCM wards is expected and a clinical psychologist at Norwich Hospital observed, "PCM patients function more autonomously and level of functioning has improved visably. This has taken the form of a reduction of hallucinations, improved behavior, and reduction of behavioral patterns that were deemed inappropriate but have been habitual for years. Patients who initially exhibited severe behavioral problems have dropped and modified these patterns once involved in PCM wards. For example, tantrum behavior is fairly quickly extinguished, demanding-dependent behavior yields to more independent functioning. One of the most obvious changes on the PCM wards is that of increased communication and interaction. Peer-peer interaction has increased significantly."[10]

A few examples of successes with individual patients will highlight the strides that can be made using this system of care. A 65-year-old suffered from incapacitating auditory hallucinations and fears. She is currently a coleader of the Patients' Advisory Council.

A 65-year-old has depressive episodes with psychotic features, is fearful of decompensating and afraid to go out of the facility. Since PCM she has begun to work in the commisary, has been shopping, and dines out with friends.

A 94-year-old had refused to have a cataract operation. After the ward got a cat, she approached her family group leader (cluster leader) and asked to get "her eyes fixed" so she could see the color of the cat.

An 80-year-old who had refused to move from her wheelchair now walks with a walker.

A 78-year-old refused to leave her room and now acts as hostess for newcomers to the floor. Interest groups, led by aides, take place regularly on the floor. Activities personnel teach group leadership techniques. Weekly mini-team meetings (aides, social worker, recreation worker and nurse) review problems and direction at the floor level as primary helpers seek assistance with any resident of their cluster.

As one patient said when asked what PCM meant to her, "An opportunity to think for myself, to make my own decisions."

SUMMARY OF SPECIAL FEATURES

The Personalized Care Model is a system marked by a number of features that make possible personalization in the planning and treatment process, humanization with respect to staff attitudes and environmental conditions, and eventuation of potential-oriented expectations; all of which impact significantly on the mental well-being and physical status of the institutionalized elders.

The system:

is dynamic in nature and adapts to the changing environment

facilitates attitudinal, emotional and behavioral change

has its foundations in cultural anthropology and comparative under-standings of human behavior, order and possibilities

has a theoretical frame of reference in cultural change studies and role theory

provides a systematic approach to analyzing and integrating the total institutional environment

is holistically conceptualized

takes into consideration the whole person in a total environment

incorporates a multidisciplinary educational component

encompasses space and its utilization as an integral part of the treatment process

incorporates interpersonal relationships that personalize and humanize interaction

establishes a pattern of staff organization that facilitates implementation of the system and enables staff to establish PCM relationships

motivates staff to create and plan meaningful activities

ensures accountability on the part of the staff and continuity of care for the patient

ACTIVITY ANALYSIS FORM

Activity name: _____

Equipment needed: (be specific)

_____

_____

_____

Activity duration:

1–15 minutes	_____	45–1 hour	_____
15–30 minutes	_____	Continuous	_____
30–45 minutes	_____	Other	_____

Type of preparation: _____

_____

_____

Space required:

Small activity room	_____	Terrace area	_____
Large activity room	_____	Garden area	_____
Auditorium size	_____	Outdoor area	_____

Other area _____

Set-up required:

Chairs _____   Tables _____   Other _____

Number of participants required:

Men _____   Women _____   Other _____

Leadership required:

General recreation

leadership	_____	Drama therapist	_____
Art specialist	_____	Outside specialist	_____
Music specialist	_____	Other	_____
Dance therapist	_____		

What is the role of the leader? _____

_____

Skills and abilities:

Sensory-motor requirements:

What type of movement is involved?

Standing	_____	Walking	_____	Pushing	_____
Sitting	_____	Running	_____	Pulling	_____
Bending	_____	Skipping	_____	Stretching	_____
Turning	_____	Jumping	_____	Throwing	_____
Twisting	_____	Bopping	_____	Hitting	_____
Other	_____				

What parts of the body are needed for movement?

Arms _____   Fingers _____   Legs _____

Toes _____   Hands _____   Head _____
Neck _____   Other _____

Is there any coordination of body part required?
                Yes _____   No _____

If so, which parts are required?
_____

What are the primary senses required for the activity?
Vision _____ Hearing _____ Touch _____ Taste _____ Smell _____

How much of each sense will be needed?
_____

Which sense will be used the most? List in order of usage.
1. _____   3. _____   5. _____
2. _____   4. _____

Which of the following physical requirements will be necessary?
Eye-hand coordination _____   Speed   _____
Muscular strength   _____   Dexterity   _____
Flexibility   _____

Cognitive skills:

What cognitive skills are required?

Skill:	None:	Some:	Much:
Memorization			
Learning ability			
Retention			
Long-term			
Short-term			
Attention span			
Concentration			
Strategy			
Understanding			
goals of activity			
rules of activity			
procedure(s) of activity			
Verbal communication			
Non-verbal communication			
Intellectual skills			
Reading			
Writing			
Spelling			
Math			
Communication other than written language			
Music			
Picture objects			
Other symbols			
Sizes and shapes			
Numbers			
Concrete thinking			

Abstract thinking   _____
Auditory sounds   _____
Other   _____

Affective skills

What are the emotional demands of the activity?

Joy/happiness _____	Sadness _____	Anger _____
Guilt _____	Frustration _____	Agitation _____
Fear _____	Apathy _____	Anxiety _____
Other _____		

Social skills

Number of required participants: _____

Type of social communication required for activity:

Verbal _____	Non-verbal _____	Visual _____
Hearing _____	Touching _____	

Interactive pattern required for activity:

Intra-individual _____	Unilateral _____
Extra-individual _____	Multilateral _____
Aggregate _____	Intra-group _____
Inter-individual _____	Inter-group _____

What is the structure of the activity?

No structure _____   Some structure _____   Highly structured _____

What is the proximity of the patients?

Close together _____   Far apart _____   Can be seen _____
Cannot be seen _____

What is the nature of the activity?

Competitive _____ (individual)	Competitive _____ (team)	Cooperative _____

What are the genders required for the activity?

Women only _____   Men only _____   Men and women _____

Are there functional skills required?
(Activities of daily living)

Dressing _____   Undressing _____   Other_____

PROGRAM EVALUATION FORM

ACTIVITY: _____

ACTIVITY LEADER: _____ DATE: _____

EVALUATION AREAS	YES	NO	ACTION RECOMMENDED
PROGRAM PREPARATION:			
1. Worker uses appropriate channels to inform residents of program time, place, purpose.			
2. Worker has sufficient equipment supplies, etc. for activity.			
3. Worker has arranged for transport of patients to activity.			
4. Worker has set up equipment and space to best advantage for program.			
5. Worker has several possibilities in event that patients are not responsive to scheduled activity.			
6. Other: _____			
LEADERSHIP:			
1. Worker shows awareness of patient's interests.			
2. Worker shows awareness of patient's skills. (Delegates activity tasks accordingly)			
3. Worker shows awareness of patient's disabilities and functional deficits (adapts equipment, modifies activity situation accordingly)			
4. Worker attempts to motivate withdrawn patients.			
5. Worker provides structure for confused and memory-impaired. environmental verbal mediation			
6. Worker attempts to make regular contact with all patients in the activity area. (i.e. either by verbal or non-verbal techniques)			

EVALUATION AREAS	YES	NO	ACTION RECOMMENDED
7. Worker encourages patient interaction.			
8. Worker fosters group awareness.			
9. Worker is responsive to needs of individual patients.			
10. Worker picks up on cues of patients.			
11. Worker adequately deals with disruptive or inappropriate behaviors.			
12. Worker deals adequately with agitated behavior.			
13. Worker provides instruction and guidance as needed.			
14. Worker is able to assess group "mood." (i.e. energy level, attention span, receptivity, and modify activities accordingly)			
15. Worker fosters independence in patients whenever possible.			
16. Worker shows an awareness and appropriate use of therapeutic recreation techniques.			
17. Worker is flexible resourceful imaginative			
18. Other: _____ _____ _____			
STAFF TO STAFF INTERACTION			
1. Worker has informed on-unit staff of programming.			
2. Worker is in communication with other staff:			
a. to find out about patient's non-activity behavior.			
b. re significant changes in medical and or psychological condition.			
c. to share information about patient in activities with on-unit staff.			
3. Other: _____ _____ _____			

EVALUATION AREAS	YES	NO	ACTION RECOMMENDED
EVALUATOR'S SIGNATURE: _____			
TITLE: _____			

ACTIVITIES PREFERENCE QUESTIONNAIRE AND ASSESSMENT

Name: _____ Sex: _____ Room: _____
Date of birth: _____ Date admitted: _____
Country of origin: _____ Years in U.S.: _____
Religion: _____ Education: _____
Occupation: _____

HEALTH STATUS

Mental status: _____ Hearing: _____ Vision: _____
Speech: _____ Ambulation: _____
Appearance: _____
Disabilities affecting participation: _____
Communication skills: Verbal: _____ Non-verbal: _____
Un-responsive: _____ Comments: _____
Motor coordination: Fine: _____ Gross: _____
Comments: _____
Possible interaction level: Small group: _____
Large group: _____ One to one: _____
Comments: _____

FAMILY BACKGROUND

Marital status: _____ Offspring: _____
Contact with family and/or friends: _____

FORMER INTERESTS

PLEASE LIST ANY INTERESTS YOU HAD BEFORE ENTERING THE HOME.

Music: _____ Social: _____ Creative: _____ Crafts: _____
Intellectual: _____ Athletic: _____ Other: _____
Spectator activities:
Concerts: _____ Plays: _____ Movies: _____
Dance: _____ Other: _____
Volunteer experience: _____
Participation in community and/or political organizations:

PLEASE INDICATE THE TYPES OF ACTIVITIES YOU THINK YOU WOULD EN-
JOY AT THIS FACILITY.

Arts and crafts:
Knitting: _____ Crocheting: _____ Sewing: _____
Painting: _____ Needlework: _____ Other: _____

Reading:
Fiction: _____ Non-fiction: _____ History: _____
Nature: _____ Biography: _____ Travel: _____

Newspaper: _____ Magazines: _____ T.V.: _____
Radio: _____ Other: _____

Writing:
Do you like to write? _____ Stories: _____ Poetry: _____
Articles: _____ Book reviews: _____ Other: _____

Games:
Cards (specify): _____ Shuffleboard: _____ Bingo: _____
Table games: _____ Other: _____

Arts Programs:
Music Appreciation: _____ Choral group: _____ Drama group: _
What kind of music do you like?
Classical: _____ Opera: _____ Country: _____
Religious: _____ Popular: _____ Other: _____
Do you play an instrument? _____ What kind? _____
Do you like to sing? _____ Do you act? _____

Other Programs:
Adult education: _____ Current events: _____
Documentary movies: _____ Feature movies: _____
Fitness fun: _____ Cooking class: _____
Horticulture: _____ Religious study group: _____
Other: _____

Religious programs:
Sabbath services: _____ Rabbi class: _____ Mass: _____
Other: _____

Resident volunteer corps:
Recreation planning committee: _____
Religious committee: _____ Activity assistant: _____
Librarian: _____ Clerical help: _____
Mail delivery: _____ Resident council: _____
Other: _____

Family member(s) comment: (when available)
_____
_____
_____

Family member signature: _____
Relationship to resident: _____
Resident signature: _____

Activity leader's signature: _____
Interview date: _____

INDIVIDUALIZED ACTIVITIES PROGRAM SCHEDULE

Resident name: _____ Admission date: _____ Location: _____

Below is a schedule of activities *you* have expressed an interest in attending. Please keep this form handy to help you become more easily acquainted with the times and places of these activities.

	Monday	Tuesday	Wednesday	Thursday	Friday	Saturday	Sunday
9:30							
10:30							
1:30							
2:30							
3:30							
6:30							

RESIDENT CARE PLAN AND AUDIT REVIEW SYSTEM

Building: _____ Floor: _____ Activity: _____

Resident Name:	Room:	Date:	Resident Care Plan (last date)	Team Meeting	Activity Approval	Activity Quest.	Activity Leader Initial

SUGGESTED ACTIVITIES

ADAPTIVE SPORTS

A. Bowling
B. Basketball
C. Beanbag Toss

Goals of Activity:
1. To promote socialization and peer interaction.
2. To improve eye-to-hand coordination.
3. To enhance self-esteem.
4. To improve functioning of the cardiovascular system.
5. To improve muscle coordination.
6. To provide competition in a group structure.

General Procedures:
1. Sit residents in a circle so that everyone is facing each other.
2. Before playing, demonstrate how each game is played so that the residents will understand what is expected of them.
3. Explain the rules of the game.
4. Explain and demonstrate how to hold the ball or beanbag.
5. Explain and demonstrate how to throw the ball or bag.
6. Provide verbal encouragement.
7. Provide constant praise for efforts and accomplishments.

A. Bowling
   Object of game: To knock down all ten pins.
   Number of chances: two per player.
   Scoring: Add the first number of pins knocked down to the second number
            of pins knocked down.
   Specific procedures:
   1. Set up ten pins in the shape of a pyramid at a distance appropriate to the functioning level of the resident.
   2. Give the ball to the resident.
   3. Demonstrate how to hold the ball and throw it.
   4. Get the resident to throw the ball, knocking down as many pins as possible.

B. Basketball (floor basket or adjustable basket can be used)
   Object of game: To get the ball into the basket.
   Number of chances: three per player.
   Scoring: Add the number of shots in each basket. Each shot is worth two
            points.
   Specific Procedures:
   1. Set the basket at a distance appropriate to the functioning level of the resident.
   2. Explain and demonstrate how to hold and throw the ball through the basket.
   3. Have resident throw the ball through the basket.

C. Beanbag* Toss (a basket or board with holes can be used)
   Object of game: To throw the beanbags one at a time through the holes
                   worth the most points.
   Number of chances: five per player.
   Scoring: Add the number values of the holes which the resident tossed the
            bag through.
   Specific Procedures:
   1. Set the beanbag board** at a distance appropriate to the functioning level
      of the resident.
   2. Explain and demonstrate how to hold and throw the beanbags.
   3. Get resident to throw the beanbags one at a time through the holes.

* Beanbags can be made by the residents as an arts and crafts project.
**Beanbag boards can be painted with different faces.

MUSICAL GAMES

A. Name that Tune
B. Tic-Tac-Tune
C. S-I-N-G-O

Goals of Activity:
1. To have a pleasurable and satisfying experience.
2. To promote socialization and peer interaction.
3. To increase auditory awareness, perception and memory.
4. To promote a competitive experience in a nonthreatening and enjoyable environment.

General Procedures:
1. Sit residents either in a circle or in a semi-circle around the piano or stereo or
   cassette player.

Materials Needed:
1. Instrument such as a piano or guitar.
2. A stereo or cassette player if no instrument is available.
3. Songbook or records.
4. Chalk and blackboard or poster board and magic markers.

A. Name that Tune
   Object of game: To guess the most number of songs.
   Number of chances: Varies

   Scoring: The resident or team which guesses the most number of songs wins
            the game.

   Specific Procedures:
   Non-competitive:
   1. Play the melody or part of the theme of the song.
   2. Ask the resident to guess the name of the song.
   3. After guessing the song title, sing the song together as a group or solo if
      the resident desires.

Competitive:
1. Divide the residents into two teams.
2. Play the melody, but ask only one team to guess the title. If they name the tune, give them one point.
3. The activity leader should write the score on a blackboard or large piece of oak tag. Excitement over scoring adds to the competitiveness of the game.
4. Sing the song through with the entire group.
5. Repeat this procedure with each team. Continue back and forth until one team accumulates ten points.
6. The length of the game is up to the group leader.

Scoring:

Team A	Team B
1111 1	111

B. Tic-Tac-Tune
   Object of game: To get tic-tac-toe by naming the titles of the songs.
   Number of chances: Varies.
   Scoring: The resident or team which guesses the most number of songs wins.

   Specific Procedures:
   1. Draw a tic-tac-toe board on a large piece of oak tag.
   2. Fill in each blank space with the title of a song.
   3. Position the residents so that the board is clearly visible to all.
   4. Choose a song on the board at random and play the song.
   5. Have the residents guess which song is being played and ask them to locate the name of the song on the board.
   6. Mark the song guessed with an "X."
   7. If teams are used, assign an "X" to one team and an "O" to the other.
   8. Sing each song together.
   9. The team or resident with Tic-Tac-Tune wins the game.

C. S-I-N-G-O (See Illustration on following page)
   Object of game: To complete the S-I-N-G-O card as you would a Bingo card.
   Number of chances: Varies.
   Scoring: The first resident or team to complete a line designated by the leader wins the S-I-N-G-O game.

   Specific procedures:

   1. Pass out pre-printed or xeroxed S-I-N-G-O cards with the names of songs printed in each box.
   2. Play the melody of each song until the resident guesses the song.
   3. Have the resident mark off the name of the song on the proper box of the card.
   4. Sing the song together after each song title is guessed.

*S-I-N-G-O cards can be prepared with the names of songs from different periods or years. Discussion groups can also be held around the themes of the songs.

S	I	N	G	O
DAISY DAISY	CLEMEN-TINE	LITTLE BROWN JUG	BABY FACE	TUXEDO JUNCTION
BLUE MOON	BILL BAILY	TILL THEN	LET ME CALL YOU SWEET-HEART	BYE-BYE BLACK-BIRD
I WANT TO BE HAPPY	CAROLINA	FREE	MAME	BOOGIE WOOGIE BUGLE BOY
TEA FOR TWO	PEG OF HEART	SMILE	SWANEE RIVER	MOON OVER MIAMI
YOU ARE MY SUNSHINE	WORKING ON THE RAILROAD	WHEN YOU WERE SWEET SIXTEEN	APRIL SHOWERS	SHUFFLE OFF TO BUFFALO

REFERENCE NOTES

1. Fred S. Greenblatt, *Drama with the Elderly: Acting at Eighty* (Springfield Illinois: Charles C. Thomas, 1985).

CHAPTER 1

1. Richard Kraus, *Recreation Today: Program Planning and Leadership* (New York: Appleton-Century Crofts, 1966), p. 9.
2. James F. Murphy, *Concepts of Leisure: Philosophical Implications* (Englewood Cliffs: Prentice-Hall, Inc., 1974), p. 79.
3. J. Tillman Hall, *School Recreation: Its Organization, Supervision and Administration* (Dubuque, Iowa: William Brown Company, 1966), p. 14.
4. James F. Murphy, quoting Clyde R. White, "Social Class Difference in the Uses of Leisure," *American Journal of Sociology* 61 (September 1955): 145–50.
5. Elliot Avedon, *Therapeutic Recreation Services: An Applied Behavioral Approach* (Englewood Cliffs: Prentice-Hall, Inc., 1974), p. 48.
6. *Ibid.*, p. 53.
7. Paul Haun, *Recreation: A Medical Viewpoint* (New York: Teachers College Press, 1971), pp. 55–56.
8. Edith Ball, "The Meaning of Therapeutic Recreation," *Therapeutic Recreation Journal* 4 (1970): 17–18.
9. Thomas Collingwood, "Therapeutic Recreation's Relevance to the Rehabilitative

179

Process," *Therapeutic Recreation Annual: National Recreation and Park Society*, Vol. III. (1971) p. 28.

10. *Ibid.*, p. 28.
11. Paul Haun, *Ibid.*, p. 54.
12. Thomas Collingwood, *Ibid.*, p. 30.
13. Gerald S. O'Morrow, *Therapeutic Recreation A Helping Profession* (2nd. ed.) (Reston, Virginia: Prentice-Hall, Inc., 1980), p. 5.
14. Ann Cronin Mosey, *Activities Therapy* (New York: Raven Press, 1973), p. 11.
15. *Ibid.*, p. 12.
16. *Ibid.*, p. 12.
17. *Ibid.*, p. 2.
18. *Ibid.*, p. 2.
19. Elliot Avedon, *Ibid.*, p. 21.
20. *Ibid.*, p. 21.

CHAPTER 2

1. *Random House Dictionary*, Jess Stein, ed., (1966), New York.
2. Elliot Avedon, *Ibid.*, p. 5.
3. Ronald P. Reynolds and Gerald S. O'Morrow, *Problems, Issues and Concepts in Therapeutic Recreation* (Englewood Cliffs: Prentice-Hall, Inc., 1985), p. 13.
4. *Ibid.*, p. 13.
5. Charles C. Bucher and Richard I. Bucher, *Recreation for Today's Society* (Englewood Cliffs: Prentice-Hall, Inc., 1974), p. 70.
6. Ronald Reynolds and Gerald O'Morrow, *Ibid.*, p. 15.
7. *Ibid.*, p. 15.
8. Gerald O'Morrow, *Therapeutic Recreation, A Helping Profession* p. 105.
9. *Ibid.*, p. 105.
10. *Ibid.*, p. 105.
11. *Ibid.*, p. 111.
12. Reynolds, R. P. and O'Morrow, G. S. *Problems, Issues and Concepts in Therapeutic Recreation* (Englewood Cliffs: Prentice-Hall, 1985.) quoting University of Minnesota and Work Progress Administration Reports of the First College Conference on Training Recreation Leaders (Minnesota: University of Minnesota, 1937), p. 25–26.

CHAPTER 3

1. Howard Danford, *Creative Leadership in Recreation* (Boston: Allyn and Bacon, 1964), p. 55.
2. *Ibid.*, p. 55.
3. Paul Haun, *Recreation: A Medical Viewpoint*, p. 60–61.
4. Ball, "The Meaning of Therapeutic Recreation," *Therapeutic Recreation Journal*, 4:1 (1970) pp. 17–18.

5. "Philosophical Position Statement," *National Therapeutic Recreation Society* (Alexandria, Virginia: 1982) p. 1.

6. *Ibid.*, p. 1.

7. Phyllis M. Foster, "Activities: A necessity for Total Health Care of the Long-Term Care residents," *Activities, Adaptation and Aging* 3(3) pp. 17–23. (Spring, 1983): 18.

CHAPTER 4

1. Elliot Avedon, *Therapeutic Recreation Services*, p. 106.

2. *Ibid.*, p. 107 quoting R. E. Carlson, T. R. Deppe and J. R. Mclean, *Recreation in American Life* (Belmont: Wadsworth Publishing Co., 1967), pp. 357–78; H. G. Danford, *Creative Leadership in Recreation*, (Boston: Allyn and Bacon, 1964), pp. 122–134; V. Frye and M. Peters, *Therapeutic Recreation* (Harrisburg, Pa: Stackpole Books, 1972), pp. 165–166; R. G. Kraus, *Recreation Today: Program Planning and Leadership* (New York: Appleton-Century Crofts, 1966), pp. 249–53; H. D. Meyer and C. K. Brightbill, *Recreation Administration* (Englewood Cliffs: Prentice-Hall, Inc., 1956), pp. 345–52; J. Pomeroy, *Recreation for the Physically Handicapped* (New York: The Macmillan Co., 1964), pp. 71–74. L. S. Rodney, *Administration of Public Recreation* (New York: The Ronald Press, 1964), pp. 204–206.

3. Howard Danford, *Creative Leadership in Recreation* (Boston: Allyn and Bacon, 1965), p. 107–108.

4. Murphy, *Concepts of Leisure*, p. 105 quoting British Travel Association, University of Keel, Pilot National Recreation Survey, Report Number 1, July 1967.

5. *Ibid.*, p. 106 quoting Joel E. Gerstl, "Leisure Taste and Occupational Milieu," *Social Problems*, (Summer, 1961).

6. Elliot Avedon, *Ibid.*, p. 111.

7. *Ibid.*, p. 21.

8. *Ibid.*, p. 123.

CHAPTER 5

1. Elliot Avedon, *Therapeutic Recreation Services*, p. 209.

2. *Ibid.*, p. 176.

3. David Arenberg; Laird Cermak; James I. Fozard; Leonard Poon and Larry W. Thompson; editors, *New Directions in Memory and Aging: Proceedings of the George A. Taland Memorial Conference* (Hillsdale, New Jersey: Lawrence Eilbaum Associates, 1980) p. 116.

4. Elliot Avedon, *Therapeutic Recreation Services*, p. 162–170. Reprinted with permission of Prentice-Hall, Inc.

5. United States Department of Health, Education and Welfare, *Activities Supervisor's Guide: A Handbook for Activity Supervisors in Long-Term Care Facilities* (Washington D.C.: Government Printing Office, December 1972), p. 8.

CHAPTER 6

1. Patricia Farell and Hubert Lundergren, *Process of Recreation Programming: Theory and techniques* (New York: John Wiley and Sons, 1978) p. 207.
2. Carole Ann Peterson and Scout Lee Gunn, *Therapeutic Recreation Program Design: Principles and Procedures* 2nd edition, (Englewood Cliffs: Prentice-Hall Inc., p. 137.
3. *Ibid.*, p. 143.
4. David Austin, *Therapeutic Recreation Processes and Techniques* (New York: John Wiley and Sons, 1982), p. 170.
5. Peterson and Gunn, *Therapeutic Recreation Program Design*, p. 144.
6. *Ibid.*, 144.
7. *Ibid.*, 145.
8. David Austin, *Ibid.*, p. 171.
9. *Ibid.*, p. 171.
10. *Ibid.*, p. 172.
11. Farell and Lundergrun, *Ibid.*, p. 216.
12. *Ibid.*, p. 217.
13. Danford, *Creative Leadership in Recreation*, p. 348.
14. Farell and Lundergrun, *Processes of Recreation Programming*, p. 213.
15. John Hutchinson, *Principles of Recreation* (New York: The Ronald Press, 1951) p. 253.
16. Farell and Lundergrun, *Ibid.*, p. 222, 229.
17. Danford, *Creative Leadership in Recreation*, p. 351.
18. Jay Shivers, *Recreation Leadership* (New Jersey: Princeton Book Company, 1980), p. 224.
19. *Ibid.*, p. 224.
20. *Ibid.*, p. 224.

CHAPTER 7

1. Danford, *Creative Leadership in Recreation*, p. 79.
2. Hall, *School Recreation: Its Organization, Supervision, and Administration*, p. 27.
3. Richard Kraus, Gay Carpenter and Barbara Bates, *Recreation and Supervision*, 2nd edition, (Philadelphia: W. B. Saunders Company, 1981), p. 11 quoting Keith Davis, *Human Relationships at Work* (New York: McGraw Hill Company, 1967), pp. 96–97.
4. Danford, *Creative Leadership in Recreation*, p. 80.

5. Danford, *Ibid.*, quoting Ralph M. Stodghill, "Personal factors association with leadership: a survey of the literature," *Journal of Psychology* (January, 1948): 64.

6. Hubert Bonner, *Group Dynamics: Principles and Applications* (New York: The Roland Press, 1959), p. 169.

7. Shivers, *Recreational Leadership*, p. 88 quoting F. E. Fiedler, *A Theory of Leadership Effectiveness* (New York: McGraw Hill Book Company, 1967)

8. *Ibid.*, p. 89.

9. *Ibid.*, p. 89.

10. Michael S. Olmsted, *The Small Group*, 5th printing (New York: Random House Inc., 1959) p. 39 quoting Ronald Lippett and Ralph K. White, "An Experimental Study of Leadership and Group Life," readings in *Social Psychology*, revised edition, Guy Swanson, Theeodore Newcomb and Eugene Hartely, editors, (New York: Henry Holt and Co., 1952), p. 340.

11. Fred Greenblatt, *Drama with the Elderly*, (Springfield, Illinois: Charles C. Thomas, 1985), p. 3 quoting Dr. Dennis Waitely, *The Psychology of Winning: Positive Self Image*, Tape No. 3 (Chicago: Nightingale-Conant Corp., 1978)

12. Norman Cameron, *Personality Development and Psychopathology; A Dynamic Approach* (Boston: Haughton Mifflin Co., 1963), p. 347.

13. Shivers, *Recreational Leadership*, p. 125.

14. Jack Botwinick, *Aging and Behavior* (New York: Springer Publishing Co., 1973), p. 235 quoting I. Hulicka and J. Grossman, "Age group comparisons for the use of mediators in a paired-associate learning," *Journal of Gerontology*, (1967): 22.

15. Jay Shivers, *Ibid.*, p. 187.

CHAPTER 8

1. This chapter was written by and used with permission of Dr. Miriam Lahey, Acting Chairman, Department of Physical Education, Recreation and Dance, Lehman College, The Bronx, New York.

2. G. Niederehe and E. Fruge, "Dementia and family dynamics: clinical research issues," *Journal of Geriatric Psychiatry* 17 (1985): 21–56.

3. M. Roth, "Some strategies for tackling the problems of senile dementia and related disorders within the next decade," *Danish Medical Bulletin* 32 (Suppl. 1), (1985): 92–111.

4. M. K. Hansan, N. L. Slack and R. P. Mooney, "Diagnosis and treatment of Alzheimer's disease," *West Virginia Medical Journal* 79 (1983): 98–102.

5. C. Eisdorfer and D. Cohen "Diagnostic criteria for primary neuronal degeneration of the Alzheimer's type," *The Journal of Family Practice* 11 (1980): 553–557.

6. R. N. Butler, R. W. Besdine and J. A. Brody "Senility reconsidered: treatment possibilities for mental impairment in the elderly," *JAMA* (1980): 244, 259–263.

7. J. T. Coyle, D. L. Price and M. R. Delong "Alzheimer's disease: A disorder of cortical cholinergic innervation," *Science*, 1983, p. 219, 1184–1190.

8. J. A. Brody "An epidemiologist views senile dementia—facts and fragments," *American Journal of Epidemiology* 115 (1982): 155–162.

9. M. H. Schneck, B. Reisberg and S. H. Ferris "An overview of current concepts of Alzheimer's disease," *American Journal of Psychiatry* 139 (1982): 162–173.

10. M. H. Simank and K. J. Strickland "Assisting families in coping with Alzheimer's disease and other related dementias with the establishment of a mutual support group," *Journal of Gerontological Social Work* 9(2), (1985): 49–59.

11. Carl Eisdorfer, reported in J. Kohn, "The Issue of Alzheimer's care and treatment," *Canadian Medical Association Journal* 132 (1985): 865–870.

12. C. Rogers, *Carl Rogers on Encounter Groups* (New York: Harper and Row, 1970).

13. L. J. Novick, "Senile patients need diverse programming," *Geriatrics*, 1982.

14. Gail Weinstein, "Impact of Activities on Wandering of Nursing Home Alzheimer's Patients," (Master's Thesis, Lehman College, City University of New York, 1985).

15. J. Panella and F. H. McDowell *Day Care for Dementia* (White Plains, New York: Burke Rehabilitation Center, 1983).

16. K. Phillips, "Effectiveness of category-label primes on anagram-task performance of Alzheimer's patients," (Master's thesis, Lehman College, City University of New York, 1985).

17. R. Katzman, T. Brown, P. Fuld, A. Peck, R. Schechter, and H. Schimmel "Validation of short orientation-memory concentration test of cognitive impairment," *American Journal of Psychiatry* (1983): 140, 6.

18. C. Eisdorfer, reported in J. Kohn "The issue of Alzheimer's care and treatment," p. 876–870.

19. P. E. Davis and S. J. Mumford "Cued recall and the nature of the memory disorder in dementia," *British Journal of Psychiatry* 144 (1984):383–386; H. Diesfeldt "The importance of encoding instructions and retrieval cues in the assessment of memory in senile dementia," *Archives of Gerontology and Geriatrics* (1984); 3, 51–57.

20. C. K. Cassel "Research in nursing homes: ethical issues," *Journal of the American Geriatric Society* 33 (1985): 795–799.

21. W. James *Principles of Psychology* (New York: Henry Holt, 1890).

22. C. G. Jung, editor, *Man and His Symbols* (New York: Doubleday, 1964).

23. R. Nadeau "Using the visual arts to expand personal creativity," *Using the Creative Arts in Therapy* B. Warren, editor, (Cambridge, Mass: Brookline Books, 1984).

24. E. Streitfeld, Lecture, "Art with Alzheimer's Patients," (Lehman College, City University of New York, May 1986).

25. Nadeau, *Ibid.*

26. I. Bergman, *Ingmar Bergman, Essays in Criticism* S. M. Kaminsky, editor, (New York: Oxford University Press, 1975).

27. S. Arieti *Creativity* (New York: Basic Books, 1976).

28. Gail Weinstein (Master's thesis, Lehman College)
29. R. Nadeau, B. Warren, editor, *Creative Arts in Therapy*
30. S. Arieti, *Ibid.*
31. R. Berne, *Transactional Analysis in Psychotherapy* (New York: Grove Press, 1961)
32. Streitfeldt, Lecture, "Art with Alzheimer's Patients."

CHAPTER 9

1. O'Morrow, *Administration of Activities Therapy Service* (Springfield Illinois: Charles C. Thomas, 1966), p. 204.
2. *Volunteer and Activity Service Corps Handbook* (Washington D.C.: American Nursing Home Association, 1972) p. III
3. *Ibid.*, p. 3.
4. O'Morrow, *Ibid.*, p. 209.
5. *Volunteer and Activity Service Corps Handbook, Ibid.*, p. 9.
6. O'Morrow, *Ibid.*, p. 216.
7. *Volunteer and Activity Service Corps Handbook, Ibid.*, p. 11.
8. O'Morrow, *Ibid.*, p. 221.
9. *Volunteer and Activity Service Corps Handbook, Ibid.*, p. 16.

CHAPTER 10

1. Carole Peterson and Scout Gunn, *Ibid.*, p. 213.
2. *Ibid.*, p. 218.
3. *Long-Term Care Case Mix Reimbursement Project*, The Patient Review Instrument, RUGS II Training Program. (New York: March, 1985) p. 9.
4. *Ibid.*, p. 9.
5. *Ibid.*, p. 10.
6. Steven J. Balcerzak, "Update: The New Long-Term Care Survey Process," *The Journal of Long-Term Care Administration* (Winter 1985): 106–108.
7. *Ibid.*, p. 106.

EPILOGUE

1. Alex Comfort, *A Good Age* (New York: Crown Publishers, Inc., 1976) p. 27.

BIBLIOGRAPHY

American Nursing Home Association. *Volunteer and Activity Service Corps Handbook-Organizing A Volunteer Program in the Nursing Home.* Washington, D.C.: American Nursing Home Association, Revised 1972.

Ardis, Stevens. *Fun is therapeutic: A recreation handbook to help therapeutic recreation leaders.* Springfield, Illinois: Charles C. Thomas, 1972.

Arenberg, David; Cermak, Laud; Fozard, James; Poon Leonard and Thompson, Larry W., editors, *New Directions in Memory and Aging: Proceedings of the George Taland Memorial Conference.* Hillsdale, New Jersey: Lawrence Eilbaum Associates, 1980.

Aronson, M. K. and Yatzkan, E. S., "Coping with Alzheimer's disease through support groups." *Aging,* #347, October-November 1984, pp. 3–9.

Austin, David. *Therapeutic Recreation and Techniques.* New York: John Wiley and Sons, 1982.

Balcerzak, Stephen J. "The Patient Care and Services (PaCS) Survey, Update: The New Long-Term Care Survey Process." *The Journal of Long-Term Care Administration* (Winter 1985): 106–108.

Barnes, Jonathan A. "Effects of Reality Orientation Classroom on Memory Loss, Confusion and Disorientation in Geriatric Patients." *The Gerontologist.* Vol. 14(2) (April 1974): 138–142.

Bonner, Hubert. *Group Dynamics: Principles and Applications.* New York: The Ronald Press, 1959.

Brown, Roger. *Social Psychology.* New York: The Free Press, Macmillan and Company, 1965.

Bucher, Charles and Bucher, Richard. *Recreation for Today's Society.* Englewood Cliffs, New Jersey: Prentice-Hall, Inc., 1974.

Bucher, Charles A. and Bucher, Richard D. *Recreation for Today's Society.* 2nd edition. Englewood Cliffs, New Jersey: Prentice-Hall Inc., 1984.

Butler, R. N.; Besdine, R. W.; and Brody, J. A. "Senility reconsidered: treatment possibilities for mental impairment in the elderly." *JAMA,* 244 (1980): 259–263.

Cameron, Norman. *Personality Development and Psychopathology: A dynamic approach.* Boston: Houghton Mifflin Company, 1963.

Caplow, Lindner; Harpaz, Leah; and Samberg, Sonya. *Therapeutic Dance Movement.* New York: Human Sciences Press, 1979.

Cohen, D.; Kennedy, G; and Eisdorfer, C.; "Phases of change in the patient with Alzheimer's dementia: A conceptual dimension for designing health care management." *Journal of the American Geriatrics Society* 32 (1984): 11–15.

Comfort, Alex. *A Good Age.* New York: Crown Publishers, 1976.

Corbin, Dan H. *Education for Leisure.* Englewood Cliffs, New Jersey: Prentice-Hall, Inc., 1973.

Corbin, Dan H. *Recreation Leadership.* 3rd edition, Englewood Cliffs, New Jersey: Prentice-Hall Inc., 1970.

Coyle, Grace L. *Group Experience and Democratic Values.* New York: The Woman's Press, 1947.

Curtis, J. E. *Recreation Theory and Practice.* St. Louis: C. V. Mosby Company, 1979.

Danford, Howard G. *Creative Leadership in Recreation.* Boston: Allyn and Bacon, 1965.

Davis, John E. *Clinical Applications of Recreation Therapy.* Springfield Illinois: Charles C. Thomas, Publisher, 1952.

Davis, P. E. and Mumford, S. J. "Cued recall and the nature of the memory disorder in dementia." *British Journal of Psychiatry* 144 (1984): 383–386.

Diesfeldt, H. F. A. "The importance of encoding instructions and retrieval cues in the assessment of memory in senile dementia." *Archives of Gerontology and Geriatrics,* 1984, pp. 51–57.

Diesfeldt, H. F. A. "The distinction between long-term and short-term memory in senile dementia: An analysis of free recall and delayed recognition." *Neuropsychologia,* 16, 1978, pp. 115–119.

Donahue, Wilma; Hunter, Woodey; Coons, Dorothy H; and Maurice, Helen K., editors, *Free Time-Challenge to Later Maturity.* Ann Arbor, Michigan: University of Michigan Press, 1958.

Dulles, F. R. *America Learns to Play: A History of Popular Recreation: 1607–1940.* Gloucester Mass: Peter Smith, 1959.

Edginton, Christopher; Hanson, Carole; and Compton, David. *Recreation and Leisure Programming: A Guide for Professionals.* Philadelphia: Holt, Reinhart and Winston, 1980.

Eisdorfer, C. and Cohen, D. "Diagnostic criteria for primary neuronal degeneration of the Alzheimer's type." *The Journal of Family Practice* 11 (1980): 553–557.

Farell, Patricia and Lundegren Herbert, M. *Process of Recreation Programming: Theory and Techniques.* New York: John Wiley and Sons, 1978.

Fish, Harriet U. *Activities Programs for Senior Citizens.* New York: Parker Publishing Company, 1971.

Fitzgerald, Gerald, B. *Leadership in Recreation*. New York: The Ronald Press Company, 1951.

Foster, Phyllis M. "Activities: A Necessity for Total Health Care of the Long-Term Care Resident." *Activities, Adaptation and Aging*, Volume 3(3) (Spring 1983): 17–23.

Frye, Virginia and Peters, Martha. *Therapeutic Recreation: Philosophy and Practices*. Pennsylvania: Stackpole Books, 1972.

Godby, G. *Leisure Studies and Services*. Philadelphia: W. B. Saunders and Company, 1976.

Goudsmit, J.; Marrow, C. H.; Asher, D. M.; Yangihara, R. T.; Masters, C. L.; Gibbs, C. J., Jr.; and Gajdusek, D. C.; "Evidence for and against the transmittability of Alzheimer's disease." *Neurology* 30 (1980): 945–950.

Greenblatt, Fred. *Drama with the Elderly: Acting at Eighty*. Springfield, Illinois: Charles C. Thomas, 1985.

Gunn, Scout Lee. *Basic Termination for Therapeutic Recreation and Other Action Therapies*. 4th printing. Champlain Illinois: Stripes Publishing Co., 1975.

Hall, Tillman J. *School Recreation: Its Organization, Supervision and Administration*. Dubuque Iowa: William C. Brown and Company, 1966.

Hanley, I. G. "The use of signposts and active training to modify ward disorientation in dementia." *Journal of Behavior Therapy and Experimental Psychiatry*. 12 (1981): 241–247.

Hanley, I. G. and Lusty, K. "Memory aids in reality orientation: A single-case study." *Behaviour Research and Therapy*. 22 (1984): 709–712.

Harvey, Laura. "Philosophical Considerations in programming for the older adult." *Activities, Adaptation and Aging*. Volume 2(4) (Summer 1982): 7–15.

Haun, Paul. *Recreation: A Medical Viewpoint*. New York: Teachers College Press, 1971.

Homans, George, C. *The Human Group*. New York: Harcourt, Brace and World, 1950.

Hunter, Harriet, C. "The Activity Director in a Nursing Care Facility: How does she do it?" *Activities, Adaptation and Aging* Vol. 4(4) (March 1984): 13–44.

Hutchinson, John, L. *Principles of Recreation*. New York: The Ronald Press, 1951.

Kaplan, Max. *Leisure theory and policy*. New York: John Wiley and Sons, 1975.

Kleemeir, R. W., editor. *Aging and Leisure*. New York: Oxford University Press, 1961.

Kraus, Richard. *Recreation and Leisure in Modern Society*. New York: Appleton-Century Crofts, 1971.

Kraus, Richard. *Recreation Leaders Handbook*. New York: McGraw Hill Company, 1955.

Kraus, Richard. *Recreation Today: Program Planning and Leadership*. New York: Appleton, Century Crofts, 1966.

Kraus, Richard. *Therapeutic Recreation Service: Principles and Practices*. 2nd edition, Philadelphia: W. B. Saunders Company, 1978.

Kraus, Richard and Bates, Barbara. *Recreation Leadership and Supervision*. Philadelphia: W. B. Saunders Company, 1975.

Kraus, Richard; Carpenter, Carol and Bates, Barbara. *Recreation Leadership and Supervision.* 2nd edition, Philadelphia: W. B. Saunders Company, 1981.

Kraus, Richard and Curtis, Joseph. *Creative Administration in Recreation and Parks.* 2nd edition, St. Louis: The C. V. Mosby Company, 1977.

Laker, Mark. *Nursing Home Activities for the Handicapped.* Springfield Illinois: Charles C. Thomas, Publisher, 1980.

Lauter, H. "What do we know about Alzheimer's disease today? An Overview." *Danish Medical Bulletin* 32 (Supplement 1) (1985): 1–21.

Lieber, Stanley and Fesenmaier, Daniel R. *Recreation planning and management.* State College Pennsylvania: Venture Publishing Company, 1983.

McClannahan, Lynn E. and Risley, Todd R. "Design of Living Environments for Nursing Home Residents: Recruiting Attendance at Activities." *The Gerontologist* Vol. 14(3) (June 1974): 236–240.

Miller, Dulcy B. and Barry, Jane T. "The Relationship of off Premises Activities to the Quality of Life of Nursing Home Patients." *The Gerontologist* Vol. 16 (1) Part I (February 1976): 61–64.

Miller, Norman and Robinson, Duane. *The Leisure Age: Its Challenge to Recreation.* Belmont California: Wadsworth Publishing Company, 1963.

Morris, R.; Wheatley, J.; and Britton, P. "Retrieval from long-term memory in senile dementia; cued recall revisited." *British Journal of Clinical Psychology* 22 (1983): 141–142.

Mosey, Ann C. *Activities Therapy.* New York: The Raven Press, 1973.

Murphy, James *Concepts of Leisure: Philosophical Implications.* Englewood Cliffs: Prentice-Hall, Inc., 1974.

Murphy, James F. *Leisure Service Delivery System: a Modern Perspective.* Philadelphia: Lea and Febiger, 1973.

Nash, Bryan J. *Philosophy of Recreation and Leisure.* Dubuque, Iowa: William C. Brown and Company, 1953.

Niederehe, G. and Fruge, E. "Dementia and Family Dynamics: Clinical Research Issues." *Journal of Geriatric Psychiatry* 17 (1985): 21–56.

Olmstead, Michael. *The Small Group.* 5th edition, New York: Random House, 1959.

O'Morrow, Gerald S., editor. *Administration of Activity Therapy Service.* Springfield, Illinois: Charles C. Thomas, Publisher, 1966.

O'Morrow, Gerald S. *Therapeutic Recreation, a helping Profession.* 2nd edition. Reston Virginia: Prentice-Hall, Inc., 1980.

Peterson, Carole A. and Gunn, Scout Lee. *Therapeutic Recreation Program Design.* 2nd edition, Englewood Cliffs: Prentice-Hall Inc., 1984

Portnoy, Enid P. "Aging sensory losses and communication behavior." *Activities, Adaptation and Aging* 2(1) (Fall 1981): 59–66.

Reynolds, Ronald P. and O'Morrow, Gerald S. *Problems, Issues and Concepts in Therapeutic Recreation.* Englewood Cliffs: Prentice-Hall, Inc., 1985

Ronda, James P. *Job Analysis of Recreation Leaders.* Monticello, Illinois: Vance Bibliographies, 1979.

Roth, M. "Some strategies for tackling the problems of senile dementia and related disorder within the next decade." *Danish Medical Bulletin* 32 (Suppl. 1), (1985): 92–111.

Russell, Ruth V. *Planning programs in Recreation.* St. Louis: Mosby and Company, 1982.

Schlotter, Bertha E. *Experiments in recreation with the mentally retarded; a joint project of Lincoln State school and Illinois Institute for Juvenile research.* Springfield Illinois: Department of Welfare: National Mental Health Funds, 1951.

Schneck, M. K.; Reisberg, B.; and Ferris, S. H. "An overview of current concepts of Alzheimer's disease." *American Journal of Psychiatry* 139 (1982): 165–173.

Schwenk, Mary Ann. "Reality orientation for the institutionalized aged: Does it help?" *The Gerontologist* 19 (4) (1979): 373–379.

Sessoms, Douglas H.; Meyer, Harold D.; and Brightbill, Charles K. *Leisure Services: The Organized Recreation and Park System.* 5th edition, Englewood Cliffs: Prentice-Hall, Inc., 1975.

Sessoms, Douglas H. and Stevenson, Jack L. *Leadership and Group Dynamics in Recreation Services.* Boston: Allyn and Bacon, 1981.

Shivers, Jay S. *Essentials of Recreational Services.* Philadelphia: Lea and Febiger, 1978.

Shivers, Jay S. *Leadership in Recreation Service.* New York: Macmillan Company, 1963.

Shivers, Jay S. *Leisure and Recreation Concepts: A Critical Analysis.* Boston: Allyn and Bacon, 1981.

Shivers, Jay S. *Principles and Practices of Recreation Service.* New York: Macmillan Co., 1967.

Shivers, Jay S. *Recreation Leadership: Group Dynamics and Interpersonal Behavior.* New Jersey: Princeton Book Co., 1980.

Shivers, Jay S.; Bucher, Richard D.; and Bucher, Charles A. *Recreation for Today's Society.* 2nd edition. Englewood Cliffs: Prentice-Hall Inc., 1984.

Shivers, Jay and Fait, Hollis. *Recreational Service for the Aging.* Philadelphia: Lea and Febiger, 1980.

Stein, Thomas A. and Sessoms, Douglas. *Recreation and Special Populations.* Boston: Holbrook Press, 1973.

Therapeutic Recreation Annual. Vol. VIII, 1971. National Therapeutic Recreation Society. National Recreation and Park Association.

Tillman, A. A. *The Program Book for the Recreation Professional.* Palo Alto, California: National Press Books, 1973.

United States Congress. *Alzheimer's Disease Research. Hearings, Washington G.P.O.,* 1985: 98th Congress, 2nd session, August 30-September 20, 1984.

United States Department of Health, Education and Welfare. *Activities Supervisor's Guide.* Washington, D.C.: United States Government Printing Office.

Vannier, M. *Recreation Leadership.* Philadelphia: Lea and Febiger, 1977.

Wehman, Paul., editor, *Recreation Programs for the Developmentally Disabled Person.* Baltimore: University Park Press, 1979.

Weiskopf, Don. *A guide to Recreation and Leisure.* Boston: Allyn and Bacon, 1975.

Witt, Jody; Campbell, Marilyn; and Witt, Peter. *A Manual of Therapeutic Group Activities for Leisure Education.* Washington, D.C.: Hawkins and Associates, 1979.

Woods, R. T. "Specificity of learning in reality orientation sessions: a single-case study." *Behaviour Research and Therapy* 21 (1983): 173–175.

Zarit, S. H.; Zarit, J. M.; and Reever, K. E. "Memory training for severe memory loss: Effects on senile dementia patients and their families." *The Gerontologist* 22 (1982): 373–377.

INDEX

Authoritarian program planning, 43
Autocratic leadership, 90
Avedon, Elliot, 20, 41
  on interactive processes, 61, 64, 67
  on secondary disability, 27, 48

Ball, Edith, 22, 36
Basketball, 65, 175
Beanbag toss, 175, 176
Behavior, 23, 24, 57–61, 67, 68
  changes, 26–27, 38, 77–78
  negative, 26
  and secondary disability, 48
  and self-image, 92–93
Bergman, Ingmar, 113
Berne, Eric, 115
Bonner, H., 88
Bowling, 58, 60, 175
Budget, 14, 52
  for volunteer services, 120

Cameron, Norman, 92
Case mix reimbursement, 143
Certification, 33, 35
Client assessment, 43–49, 74, 98, 130,
    131–132
  initial, 133–134, 135
Client satisfaction, 69, 101
Cognitive processes, 47, 59–60, 67, 68
Cognitively impaired, 105–115
  games for, 59–60, 110–111
  in institutions, 107–108
  safety for, 109
  statistics on, 105
Collingwood, Thomas, 22
Comfort, Alex, 153
Communication, 59, 60
  in leadership, 91–92, 103–104
Community resources, 53–54
Control groups, 77–78
Council for the Advancement of
    Hospital Recreation, 32
Creativity, 97, 103
Current practices approach to
    program planning, 42–43

Danford, Howard, 34
  on evaluation, 79
  on leadership, 86, 87
  on program planning, 42
  on sociometry, 83
Davis, Keith, 86–87
Democratic leadership, 91, 102, 104
Denial, 93, 107
Depression, 47, 60, 107
Disability
  and program planning, 32, 47
  secondary, 27, 48
Discrepancy evaluation, 73–76
  problems in, 76
Diversional activities, 66
Documentation, 14, 79, 128, 136,
    137–143, 145–151
  charting methods, 137
  goals and plans in, 139–143
  for resident care and progress, 136,
    138–139
  and RUGS system, 144–145

Education
  of activity directors, 50, 99
  background of clients, 44, 45
  curricula, 32, 33
Eisdorfer, Carl, 107, 110
Emotions, 61, 62
Ethnic backgrounds, of clients, 45–46
Evaluation, 69–85
  areas of, 83–85
  of behaviors, 58–61, 74
  of client limitations, 28, 59
  definition of, 71, 73
  of facilities, 74–75, 85
  importance of, 70–71
  of leaders, 83–84, 103
  of leisure needs, 49
  measurement tools for, 80–83, 85
  models of, 73–76
  by objectives, 80
  problems in, 69–70, 76
  in program planning, 68, 70, 76
  qualifications required for, 76–77
  by standards, 78–80